Psychiatric nursing

Psychiatric nursing

Fourth edition

Ruth V. Matheney, R.N., Ed.D.

Professor and Chairman, Department of Nursing
Nassau Community College, Garden City, N. Y.

Mary Topalis, R.N., B.S., M.A.

Chairman, Department of Nursing
Fairleigh Dickinson University, Rutherford, N. J.

The C. V. Mosby Company

Saint Louis   1965

Preface

The field of psychiatric nursing continues to undergo considerable change. Although progress is being made on many fronts, actual practice in the field continues to range from the old custodial-control concept to the dynamic approach. In addition to the increasing trend toward the dynamic base, utilizing interpersonal skills, the field is being affected by the expansion of facilities for the care of the mentally ill and a greater emphasis upon mental health. The development of day-care and night-care centers, halfway houses, mental hygiene and emergency clinics, and other facilities has changed to some extent the settings in which psychiatric patients are treated and in which psychiatric nurses function. The greater emphasis upon mental health has underlined the need for all nurses to possess some of the basic interpersonal skills developed primarily in psychiatric nursing. The report of the Joint Commission on Mental Health and Mental Illness, *Action for Mental Health,* has stimulated discussion and action and has pinpointed for the nursing profession the enormity of the task confronting it in providing adequate nursing care in the field of mental health.

Every registered nurse, regardless of the clinical area in which she functions, needs to develop certain basic interpersonal skills, and these are often easiest to acquire in a psychiatric setting where the nurse's role emphasizes such skills. Every registered nurse needs to develop certain basic skills in caring for patients with psychiatric disorders. Such skills include supporting therapy by others, using self-understanding to improve therapeutic effectiveness, conveying the desire to understand from the patient's point of view, recognizing and accepting feelings expressed, avoiding punishing patients, using the environment and social structure therapeutically, and working with others in the provision of patient care. This is not to imply that every registered nurse should be a psychiatric nursing specialist. It does imply that every registered nurse should be safe, psychologically, with "normal" and "abnormal" patients, at least to the limit that she does not damage them further, add to their psychological problems, or complicate the therapeutic effort of others. It is for this basic level that the present textbook continues to be designed.

While the text remains focused on the hard core of the problem—the hospitalized mentally ill—what is presented has much broader application. The principles apply in a variety of psychiatric settings and to patients without psychiatric problems. They apply to relationships with other members of the health team.

The book necessarily reflects the lack of a unified and accepted theory of mental health and mental illness. It rests upon empirical evidence and the scattered research that has been done. Historically, there need be no apology for this. The development of a solid theoretical basis for psychiatric nursing is a research task of major proportions and an urgent one.

References are selective rather than comprehensive. Both the beginning student and the student with a scholarly bent have been considered.

We wish to acknowledge the debt owed the many students, patients, and colleagues who have contributed so much to this book. Their number is legion, and it would be unfair to single out any one of them. We also wish to acknowledge our appreciation for the use of the facilities of the Veterans Administration Hospital in Northport, N. Y., and the facilities of Meadowbrook Hospital, East Meadow, N. Y., in staging photographs for illustrations. The facilities at Northport Veterans Administration were made available through the courtesy of Dr. Arnold A. Schillinger, Hospital Director, and the facilities at Meadowbrook Hospital were made available through the courtesy of Dr. James Collins, Medical Superintendent. Special appreciation is extended to Mrs. Helena A. Ure, Assistant Chief Nurse, Nursing Education, of the Northport Veterans Administration, and to Miss Elizabeth Schaefer, Director of Nursing, and Miss Edith M. Augustson, Associate Director, Nursing Education, both of Meadowbrook Hospital, for their generous assistance in securing illustrations. To Evelyn P. Straus we offer deep appreciation for her photographic work and the time she generously devoted to it.

Ruth V. Matheney

Mary Topalis

Contents

Psychiatric nursing

Chapter 1

Mental health:
A social problem

There are few clinical fields in nursing in which the opportunities and challenges are more interesting or prolific than in the field of psychiatric and mental health nursing. There are few clinical fields in nursing where the nurse in her comforting role is more needed. The number of patients in psychiatric institutions in need of improved nursing care is tremendous, and the opportunities to utilize creativity in devising and implementing new patterns of nursing care are widespread. Greater public acceptance of the real meaning of mental illness and deviate behavior, greater federal interest and financial assistance, increasing knowledge about human behavior, an everwidening scope of therapeutic approaches, and a greater emphasis upon interpersonal skills in nursing generally are all having a strong impact upon psychiatric nursing practice. As a result, the opportunities to actually help patients have increased markedly, and the satisfactions to be derived from psychiatric nursing have increased proportionately. Mental health and mental illness constitute a major social health problem and present therefore a major challenge to the health professions, including nursing.

Extent of the problem

Of all the health problems confronting the American public, few have such staggering proportions or such inexact treatment resources as the problem of mental illness and mental health. Almost half of all the hospital beds in the United States on any given day are occupied by psychiatric patients. At least 700,000 patients are hospitalized each day in psychiatric beds. Estimates, accuracy uncertain, have been made that at least 17,000,000 Americans need psychiatric help. Some physicians believe that half of all patients who go to private medical practitioners suffer more from psychologic and emotional problems than from physical ailments. The annual direct cost of the care of psychiatric patients has been estimated at between $1,000,000,000 and $2,000,000,000, and when in-

1

direct costs such as loss of income are included, the cost to the American public rises to $3,000,000,000 or more.

Despite these overwhelming and well-known figures, many authorities feel that the extent of actual mental illness, not to consider the question of mental health, goes well beyond these figures. Admission rates to psychiatric hospitals are influenced by many factors; the presence of psychiatric facilities, the ability of family and friends to recognize the significance of potential patient behavior, social attitudes toward psychiatric disorders, and economic status are some of the factors. With such factors influencing admission rates, many feel that the number of patients hospitalized or actually under private psychiatric care are only a surface indication of the extent of the problem.

While no exact figures are accepted by all, practically everyone in the health field agrees that mental illness and mental health constitute a major health problem, often considered the number one health problem, in the United States. There is also general agreement that we do not yet understand fully or have a solid scientific identification of the cause-effect relationships that result in psychiatric disorders. We do have a collection of theories, and the various theories do have some commonalities. Nonetheless, we can not yet identify specific causes and specific cures in the varying psychiatric syndromes. In fact, we sometimes cannot identify with exactness what the specific psychiatric syndrome may be.

In addition to the patients who receive psychiatric therapy, a number of related social problems exist that have implications for the mental health of the American public. These problems, among others, include emotionally disturbed and psychotic children, the mentally retarded, juvenile delinquency, alcoholism, drug addiction, and the emotional problems of the aging portion of our population. There can be no question that a considerable number of children have relatively serious emotional problems, and that the trained personnel and the facilities for identifying and treating such children are sadly inadequate. Estimates of the number of children involved run as high as 10 percent of all public school children. Mentally retarded adults and children with intelligence quotients of 70 or below are considered to be between 4½ and 5 million persons, approximately 3 percent of the total population. The number of children and adolescents known to police and courts for law violation is increasing at a greater rate than their proportionate population increase, and the rise in juvenile delinquency continues each year. While the incidence of alcoholism, like mental illness, is difficult to pinpoint, estimates run as high as 4½ million in the United States. Approximately 50,000 persons are considered to be narcotic addicts. In addition to the problems of organic brain disease, our aging population is subject to many difficult emotional stresses as a result of their aging process and reduced productivity and usefulness, and the percentage of our population aged 65 years or over continues to grow rapidly.

Mental health as a social problem, therefore, must rank as one of the major challenges to the health professions, including nursing.

Problems in definition

Defining clearly what constitutes *mental illness* and *mental health* is not easy. Defining health and disease is difficult, since the concept of both constantly undergoes change and development. It is usually much simpler to identify the extremely healthy and the extremely sick than to distinguish between the borderlines of either physical or mental health. Of one thing we can be certain; the absence of disease is no longer an acceptable definition of health in either the physical or emotional sense.

Mental health is even harder to define than mental illness, and the many experts who have attempted to clarify the concept do not always agree. In general, they tend to emphasize one aspect or another of what they consider to be mental health. After an extensive survey of current literature, Marie Jahoda* indicated six general approaches that are used to develop criteria for the existence or absence of mental health. These include attitudes toward self, personal growth and self-realization, internal psychologic oneness or unity, independence from social influences, adequate reality contact, and environmental mastery. While the emphasis of various experts may differ somewhat, there seems to be general agreement that a mentally healthy person has a realistic knowledge of himself and accepts himself with his strengths and weaknesses, can be genuinely concerned for others, is more directed by inner values than outer, can take care of himself without hurting others in the process, and can tolerate stress and frustration. That a single, unifying concept of health and illness does not exist in the field of mental health is not surprising—it does not exist in the field of physical health, either.

The definition of mental illness is a relative one and is usually based upon what constitutes socially accepted behavior norms. Behavior that is normal in one culture is not infrequently considered abnormal in another culture. In mental illness, again, it is the extreme that is easiest to identify, and the closer the borderline of mental health and mental disease, the more difficult the determination of the state of health. If one thinks of health as a continuum, with the extremes of health and sickness at either end, the closer one comes to the center of the line the harder it becomes to determine if a person is sick or healthy. That there are degrees of health and illness is certain, but their clear-cut definitions remain elusive. That most well persons have a sick potential and that most sick persons have a well potential is also a statement of general agreement implicit in practically all current thinking about mental health.

Despite the fact that definitions of mental illness and mental health remain somewhat elusive, existing definitions need testing in practice and continued utilization until better definitions are developed. In spite of the semantic difficulty, the medical and nursing care of those patients labeled by the social criterion of acceptable behavior norms as mentally ill constitutes an immediate problem of enormous magnitude.

---

*Jahoda, Marie: Current concepts of positive mental health, New York, 1958, Basic Books, Inc., p. 23.

Care of the mentally ill: Old pattern

There can be no objection to the statement that the care of patients with psychiatric problems has lagged well behind the care of patients with other types of health problems and also well behind the currently available knowledge of human behavior. In general, this is usually attributed to public attitudes toward mental illness, and the care provided is considered a reflection of public social concern. The historic development of the pattern for providing care for the social deviate on a psychologic basis unfortunately took such care out of the mainstream of community life and the medical and nursing professions. The result has made utilizing current knowledge more difficult.

Before the development of psychiatric hospitals, the major resource facility in psychiatric therapy, patients were often looked upon as persons under the influence of evil spirits, and the basis of therapy was either driving the devil from the patient or driving the patient from the community. Therapy was largely punitive, a concept not yet entirely dead—although its demise should have occured long since. The next step was the provision of institutions for the socially undesirable persons or misfits, where paupers, criminals, and the mentally ill were housed together. Society's lack of interest in anything except the incarceration of undesirable persons and the protection of society from them supported a widespread pattern of abuse. The beginning recognition of the fact that some of the segregated persons were actually mentally ill, coupled with the work of pioneering reformers such as Dorothea Lynde Dix, led to the acceptance of the principle of state responsibility and provision in separate institutions for the mentally ill. The shift in therapy was from a punitive approach to the era of "moral treatment", based upon kindness and consideration for the patient as a human being, along with providing the patient with an opportunity to behave like a human being. "Moral treatment" of the mentally ill actually developed first in Europe, when Dr. Philippe Pinel in France and William Tuke in England pioneered with nonrestraint and kindly treatment of patients.

Unfortunately, as a reflection of public opinion, state hospitals, which became the primary psychiatric treatment facilities in the country, were built as large institutions away from the community and away from medical and teaching facilities. Fresh air, quiet and peace were provided for patients out in the country, but such patients were also placed out of sight and out of mind. The institutions focused on custodial care and patient control, and their very size forced impersonal attitudes. The state hospital's isolated setting and size made the recruitment of qualified personnel difficult, made keeping abreast of medical developments difficult, and forced an organization that contributed to patient chronicity much more than patient recovery. The care of patients deteriorated, and the "shame of the states" has been the subject of many studies and many books.

There can be no doubt that recent years have seen many improvements

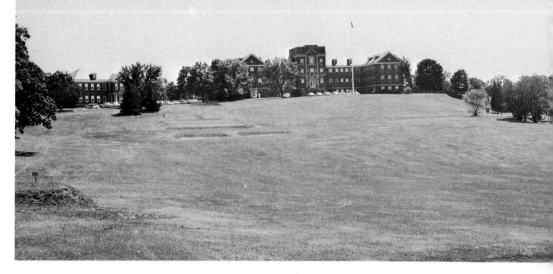

Older psychiatric hospitals are typically found in rural settings, reflecting public rejection of mentally ill patients.

in attitudes toward mentally ill patients, in the provision of social and recreational activities, in increasing the extent of the patient's responsibility for himself, and in using the psychiatric hospital environment more therapeutically. However, the well of misery has only been tapped. For each small step taken, there are many giant steps to be taken. Eighty percent of all psychiatric patients are still in state hospitals where the physical facilities, traditions, location, organization, and financing and staffing patterns make the use of modern therapeutic techniques extremely difficult. In addition to the mental patients housed in state hospitals, they are found in three other types of facilities: the Veterans Administration hospitals, small private hospitals, and psychiatric units in general hospitals.

Care of the mentally ill: New pattern

Although slowly, changes are taking place that promise real improvement for the care of the mentally ill. Current thinking and planning for mental health and the care of the mentally ill is much more comprehensive and diversified in scope than it has been in the past. The beginnings have already been indicated in the development of community, state, and regional planning bodies and in the development of new types of facilities for prevention, diagnosis, and treatment. Although there is yet much to be done, the new era has begun.

Perhaps the most significant change that has taken place has been in the area of thinking, characterized by a much broader approach to mental health and mental illness and focused on prevention, early diagnosis, treatment, and return to the community. Such thinking (and planning) envisions a wide range of services brought to the patient or potential patient when they are needed and when it is possible for him to utilize such facilities effectively.

Changes are also taking place in improving the therapeutic posture of psychiatric hospitals that are already in existence. Among the most impressive of these changes are the institution of the open-door policy, patient government, and the use of a therapeutic milieu. The open-door policy consists of open units with unlocked doors where patients accordingly assume more responsibility for their own behavior. There can be little question that the locked doors of psychiatric hospitals contributed more to the security of society than to the therapy of patients. Nonetheless, it has taken courage to open doors that have been locked for so long—despite the fact that history makes clear the value of the open-door or nonrestraint policy. While the use of patient government is not yet widespread, it has been instituted in a variety of psychiatric hospitals or units and has proved itself a valuable therapeutic adjunct. In patient government, patients participate in deciding the rules and regulations under which they live, air and settle grievances, participate in the decisions as to patients' status, help each other, and sometimes participate in therapeutic decisions. The therapeutic milieu approach to therapy includes a variety of organized efforts designed to induce patient participation in activity programs that promote improved social behavior. These can range from habit training programs aimed at bowel training, eating habits, and physical hygiene to complicated activity programs supported by individual and group therapy.

Real progress has also been made by the current resistance to increasing or expanding the large state hospitals that now exist. Planning leans toward smaller units, closer to patients and to medical centers.

Another healthy development is the slow but steady increase in psychiatric units in general hospitals. Such units, in an active treatment-centered institution, provide excellent facilities for short-term care of patients with psychiatric disorders and should contribute much to the avoidance of the development of chronic problems.

Foster family care for psychiatric patients as a substitute for hospitalization or as a transitional stage in the return to the community is not a new idea, but one which has received impetus with the recognition of the need for a broad scope of services to provide patients with necessary treatment facilities. The famous community of Gheel in Belgium has functioned in this manner successfully for many years, as patients were placed in families in the community rather than in a hospital.

Halfway houses, although not yet widespread, have been developed to help patients with the transitional period from hospital to community. They vary in the kinds of services offered, ranging from a boardinghouse type of setting to a house with intensive individual and/or group therapy offered.

Day-care and night-care centers have also been established, although these too are not yet widespread. Day-care centers provide activity and therapeutic services for patients and permit them to stay with families in the community at night. Night-care centers serve the purpose of providing a therapeutic program for patients who can continue employment. Both have the advantage of keeping the patient in contact with his community while receiving therapeutic help.

The establishment of mental health clinics was begun some time ago and has proceeded slowly. Their major problem has been overcrowding and long waiting lists. They provide diagnosis and treatment and sometimes assist with the return of patients to the community. The ultimate value of mental hygiene clinics is unquestioned, but their current value is somewhat limited by the extensive demands made upon them.

Aftercare clinics, designed to assist in patient return to the community, are also being established. Here, again, the clinics are not yet widespread, but a beginning has been made.

In some communities, emergency services on an outpatient basis are being developed, and in some places these are called walk-in clinics, open twenty-four hours a day. This type of emergency service has not been available on an outpatient basis before, and it holds real promise.

Nursing homes, with probably enough problems of their own at the present, are also a potential source of help with the milder psychiatric patient and the aging person with emotional problems. Many aged persons housed in psychiatric hospitals really belong in nursing homes. Convalescent nursing homes could also probably help with patient transition from the psychiatric hospital to the community.

Sheltered workshops also offer the possibility of a real contribution to the psychiatric therapy battery. Although the acceptance of psychiatric patients, recovered or not recovered, in sheltered workshops (where the handicapped are gainfully employed) is not widespread, some beginnings in this direction have been made, and it is anticipated that the movement will grow.

Another resource developing slowly is the establishment of expatient clubs, ranging from social groups through problem discussion to actual continuing therapy groups. Such patient clubs have been effective in areas of other health problems and with professional direction probably would be most valuable for expsychiatric patients.

Another emphasis that has developed is the stress on prevention, primary and secondary. Primary prevention is somewhat vague since it is devoted to improving mental health, and mental health, or what produces it, is not absolutely clear. Nontheless, the emphasis upon the potential mental health contribution of schools, churches, health departments, welfare departments, courts, and public recreation programs may sharpen their effectiveness. Alertness to the problem certainly should improve their contribution to secondary prevention, the early recognition and treatment of persons with emotional problems.

With the increase in the scope and variety of services available for persons with emotional problems, the health professions and the community must necessarily come to grips with the difficulty found in all health services—the need to coordinate efforts on a community level in order to provide continuity of care for individual patients.

Role of the federal government

One of the most encouraging developments in the last few years has been the interest in and the actions taken by the federal government. A national problem of the scope of the mental health problem needs a national approach. The practice of having the states primarily responsible for the care of the mentally ill ignores hard realities such as the differences in state financial incomes and the resulting variations in the ability to provide care for such patients. Mental health is a national resource and a matter of national concern.

The Mental Health Study Act of 1955 lead to the appointment of a Joint Commission on Mental Illness and Mental Health which published its famous report *Action for Mental Health* in 1961. The report identified clearly the continuing underlying problem of public rejection of the mentally ill and the key problems of man power and money needed to provide both adequate treatment and prevention. Funds made available for planning on community and regional bases, for the preparation of personnel, for research, and for construction should make substantial improvements in the mental health services available to Americans. It is only to be hoped that the expansion of services does not divert limited personnel and available funds from what the Commission identified as the hard core of the problem, the care of hospitalized mentally ill patients.

References

Angrist, Shirley S.: The mental hospital: Its history and destiny, Perspectives in Psychiatric Care 1:20-26, Dec. 1963.

American Nurses Association: Facts about nursing, New York, 1964, The Association.

Hargreaves, Anne, Warsaw, Patricia, Lewis, Edith P.: A day hospital for psychiatric patients, American Journal of Nursing 62:80-85, Sept. 1962.

Hewitt, Helon and Fatka, Nada: Social therapeutic clubs: A step toward rehabilitation, Perspectives in Psychiatric Care 1:31-37, Dec. 1963.

Jahoda, Marie: Current concepts of positive mental health, New York, 1958, Basic Books, Inc.

Joint Commission on Mental Illness and Mental Health: Action for mental health, New York, 1961, Science Editions, Inc.

Paquette, Arleen, Lafave, Hugh: Halfway house, American Journal of Nursing 64:121-124, Mar. 1964.

Surgeon General's Ad Hoc Committee on Planning for Mental Health Facilities: Planning of facilities for mental health services, Washington, D. C., Jan. 1961, United States Department of Health, Education and Welfare.

Chapter ii

The nurse in the
mental health program

In the not too distant past the psychiatric affiliation or experience provided for students of nursing was focused largely on developing an understanding of people, although trying to teach an understanding of people in a typical state hospital system may be a little difficult to understand. It seems an easier setting might have been found. In recent years more emphasis has been placed upon the student developing the ability to provide nursing care for psychiatric patients. While the changing emphasis has been occurring, changes in health problems, health services, educational patterns, and in the broad field of nursing itself have introduced considerable confusion. Exactly what constitutes psychiatric nursing is not as clear as it used to be, just as what constitutes nursing itself is not as clear as it was once assumed to be.

Nurses in psychiatric settings

Nurses and physicians, like the general public, have tended to avoid psychiatric patients, and it is to be hoped that slowly changing public attitudes will be reflected by the medical and nursing professions. There is some indication that this may occur, since both psychiatrists and psychiatric nurses find themselves granted increasing respect and acceptance by their colleagues. Psychiatrists and their colleagues in the field of psychiatry are no longer low men on the medical totem pole, and their services are in increasing demand by the public. However, the single most serious problem in the provision of care for psychiatric patients, still the most pressing problem in mental health, is the short supply of qualified manpower: physicians, nurses, psychologists, social workers, and all of the others.

While over half of all hospitalized patients occupy psychiatric beds, only 5 percent of the total number of nurses are employed in the field of psychiatric nursing. Many of these nurses are concentrated in metropolitan or urban areas in intensive treatment centers. Many of the nurses employed in state hospitals are found in administrative or teaching positions. Another major problem is the limited number of nurses in psychiatric nursing fully prepared for leadership positions at the master's or doctorate levels. While funds from the National Institute of Mental Health have been available to prepare such leadership persons since 1946, the number so prepared is hopelessly inadequate in the face of the tremendous needs that confront us. The need for psychiatric nurses is overwhelming. This need deserves definition in terms of what psychiatric nursing is, who shall do psychiatric nursing, and how varying types of personnel can best be prepared.

Psychiatric nursing: What is it?

There is no general agreement among psychiatric nursing leaders themselves as to exactly what psychiatric nursing is or what roles and functions the psychiatric nurse should assume. This is quite understandable in the light of rapid changes that are taking place both in nursing and in the care of psychiatric patients.

For many years "psychiatric" nurses (a dubious label) were considered to be those nurses who worked in settings where psychiatric patients were hospitalized. Their functions were organized around custodial care and ward management. As the emphasis in psychiatry shifted from a descriptive approach, based on syndromes of patient symptoms, to a dynamic approach, based upon the meaning of patient symptoms, a change in nursing function logically followed. Greater attention was focused upon the scientific utilization of interpersonal relationships and the use of the nurse as a person in a therapeutic sense. Later, as the social aspects of psychiatric disorders received increasing emphasis, skills in the utilization of group relationships and the manipulation of the environment, including its social organization, for therapeutic purposes were added to the needed skills. These changes have taken place at very uneven rates, and actual psychiatric nursing practice at present runs the full gamut from the old custodial-control approach to settings where nurses participate actively in individual and group patient therapy. This state of affairs has led to the objection that a nurse does not necessarily function as a psychiatric nurse even though she works in a psychiatric setting. Such an objection is legitimate.

The changing pattern of major health problems has also introduced some confusion into the concept of what constitutes psychiatric nursing. For many years the psychologic aspects of nursing were considered the exclusive property of psychiatric nursing. But with chronic diseases constituting our major killers and therefore afflicting the majority of our hospitalized patients, a change in general hospital patient needs for compassion, understanding and teaching has resulted. To meet the inevitable psychologic needs that accompany the occurrence of diseases such as cancer and heart disease has made interpersonal skill a necessary skill for the nurse on a medical or surgical floor. Increasing knowledge about the

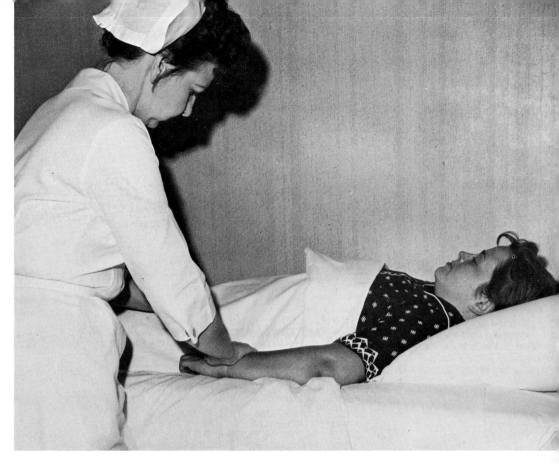

The skills emphasized in psychiatric nursing are needed by medical and surgical patients as well.

effect of hospitalization on children and the need of mothers during pregnancy and delivery for emotional support has highlighted the need for interpersonal skills on the part of the nurse in these clinical areas as well. As nursing in all areas has moved closer to psychiatric nursing in the acceptance of the need for the ability to work with and for people, the distinctions between psychiatric nursing and other fields of nursing have become more blurred. Here again in actual nursing practice, the degree of utilization of interpersonal skills in nursing varies widely and the range goes from a task oriented, get-things-done approach to a patient-centered, patient-oriented approach including full recognition of the significance of the psychologic aspects of nursing care.

An additional factor bearing on the interpretation of what constitutes psychiatric nursing is found in the newer, more comprehensive approach to the problem of mental illness and mental health, with the resultant development of newer types of facilities. Although the utilization of nurses in day-care and night-care centers, halfway houses, mental hygiene clinics and other developing facilities is quite limited as yet, the newer facilities are influencing thinking about the roles, functions, and responsibilities of

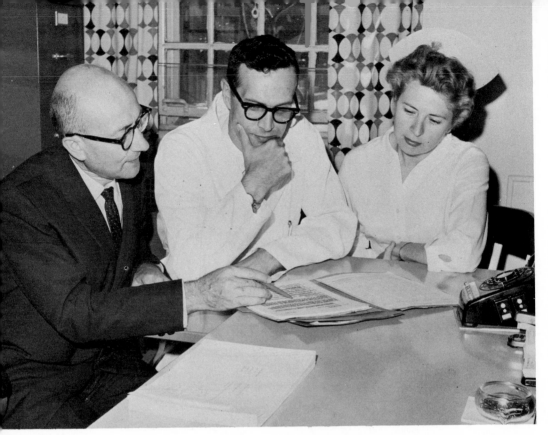

A psychologist, a psychiatrist, and a nurse confer about their respective contributions to patient care.

the nurse. In general the trend seems to be toward greater therapeutic responsibility for the nurse in one-to-one and group relationships, working on a collaborative basis with other members of the health team.

Confusing further the picture of what constitutes psychiatric nursing is the problem inherent in all nursing—the differentiation of levels of desired competency within nursing in general and also within the various clinical areas. We have graduates of basic nursing with associate degrees, baccalaureate degrees, and diplomas from schools of nursing. We have graduates with master's degrees, at least theoretically prepared for teaching, administration, consultation, and more recently expert psychiatric nursing. We also have a very few nurses prepared for psychiatric nursing at the doctorate level. Outnumbering many times all of these combined is the group of aids and attendants who comprise the largest core of personnel involved in the care of psychiatric patients. The level of roles, functions, and responsibilities of all these groups have been no more clearly defined and accepted in psychiatric nursing than in any other clinical field of nursing. Thinking ranges from the belief that all these varied groups have a place in the provision of psychiatric nursing to the belief that only a nurse with a minimum of a master's preparation for the field is competent to give "psychiatric nursing."

In the light of the preceding paragraphs, and fully aware of its limitations, the following definition of psychiatric nursing is proposed. Psychiatric nursing practice is the provision of nursing care to patients where the *major* therapeutic goal is the prevention, detection, treatment, and rehabilitation of psychiatric disorders. In providing such care, the function of the nurse is not different in nature from nursing in other clinical fields, but does differ in its *primary* focus on interpersonal one-to-one and group relationships.

Nursing and mental health

Mental health, as contrasted with mental illness, focuses upon primary and secondary prevention of mental illness. Primary prevention involves the promotion of positive mental health and secondary prevention in-

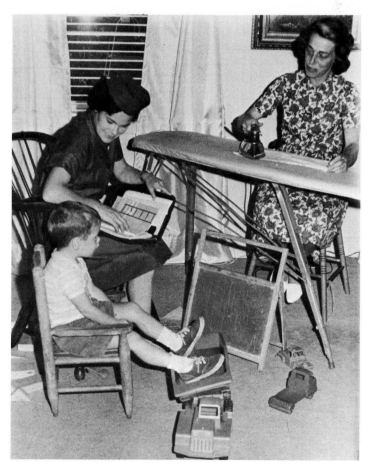

The public health nurse who visits in the home has a unique opportunity to contribute to the prevention and early detection of emotional problems. (Courtesy Nassau County Department of Health, New York.)

volves early diagnosis and treatment. One thing is certain—mental health nursing is not and cannot be the exclusive province of psychiatric nurses. There are several very practical reasons for this. From a realistic point of view, there simply are not enough psychiatric nurses to undertake the task. In addition, there is no prospect of preparing enough psychiatric nurses for such a task in the immediate future. A second practical reason is that many nurses in other clinical fields and varying specialities are already in key settings for the detection of significant signs and symptoms that could lead to early diagnosis and treatment. Public health nurses have access to families and could not only recognize and refer emotional conflicts and symptoms, but also are in a position to provide emotional support to families in many situations. Such situations include family conflicts, problem children, returning psychiatric patients, and many similar family problems. In well-baby and pediatric clinics, public health and clinic nurses are in a strategic position to make observations, to refer patients for special treatment, and to provide emotional support to parents and children. The school nurse teacher, with her invaluable contacts with children and sometimes their parents, has a rare opportunity to contribute to both primary and secondary prevention. Another nurse in a key position to make a mental health contribution is the industrial nurse. Those nurses who function in the clinical specialties of medicine, surgery, obstetrics, and pediatrics have valuable opportunities to observe, identify, and refer for help persons with emotional conflicts and symptoms. Nurses in the clinical specialities also can make a significant contribution to mental health through making the "sick" role more palatable and through helping patients with emotional support through the crises of hospitalization. Private duty nurses have the same opportunities. This is not to say that all nurses are prepared to assume the responsibilities of mental health nursing; it is only to say that in the future they must be. Mental health nursing is the responsibility of every nurse, not of psychiatric nurses alone.

References

Bermosk, Loretta S.: Preparation for psychiatric nursing in the baccalaureate program. In Education and supervision in mental health and psychiatric nursing, National League for Nursing, New York, 1963, pp. 19-26.

Gregg, Dorothy E.: The therapeutic roles of the nurse, Perspectives in Psychiatric Care 1:18-24, Jan.-Feb. 1963.

Jones, Maxwell: Psychiatric nursing is out of tune in the U.S.A., American Journal of Nursing 64:103-105, Jan. 1964.

Marchesini, Erika H. E.: The widening horizon in psychiatric nursing, American Journal of Nursing 59:978-981, July 1959.

Matheney, Ruth V.: Psychiatric nursing in the associate degree programs. In Education and supervision in mental health and psychiatric nursing, National League for Nursing, New York, 1963, pp. 27-30.

Mereness, Dorothy: The potential significant role of the nurse in community mental health services, Perspectives in Psychiatric care 1:34-39, May-June-July 1963.

Petty, John G.: Psychiatric nursing in diploma schools of nursing. In Education and supervision in mental health and psychiatric nursing, National League for Nursing, New York, 1963, pp. 31-37.

Rieman, Dwight W.: Health department nursing services for mentally ill patients and their families, Nursing Outlook **10**:450-452, July 1962.

Robinson, Alice M.: Creativity takes courage, Nursing Outlook **11**:499-501, July 1963.

Tuteur, Werner: As you enter psychiatric nursing, American Journal of Nursing **56**:72-74, June 1956.

Wolff, Isle S.: The psychiatric nurse in community mental health: A rebuttal, Perspectives in Psychiatric Care **2**:11-18, Nov. 1964.

Personality

Chapter iii

The evolution
of personality

The behavior of any given individual is an extremely complex phenomenon, and understanding its meaning is not a simple matter. Any behavior pattern is a dynamic development, with its roots in the past which have a strong influence on its present expression, and the past and the present combine to indicate future trends. Personality, of which overt behavior is one aspect, goes through successive stages of development on the road to maturity. Some understanding of the process of this development is necessary to understand behavior.

Definition

We are speaking of personality in a technical sense, and therefore must dissociate it from its common meaning. We are not referring to a person as possessing a pleasant personality, a nasty personality, or a charming personality. By personality is meant all that a person is, feels, and does, consciously and unconsciously, as manifested in interaction with his environment. Personality is not a system of traits existing solely within the capsule of a person. It is the inward organization of an individual in interaction with the outward organization of his environment, the most important parts of which are the significant persons in it. Personality is something always in the process of becoming something else, yet retaining a continuity that makes it ordinarily identifiable from situation to situation, from year to year, and from birth to death. Behavior, in both its outward and inward manifestations, is a function or expression of personality.

Motivations of behavior

What are the potentialities of any given individual as a person and what determines which potentialities shall be developed and which shall remain latent? How much *do* we know?

First, we must accept that what we know is not all, that there is more to learn than has yet been learned. The theories we now hold concerning behavior are the most adequate explanations we have yet been able to devise up to the present. However, by way of caution, we cannot use diagnostic procedures as a precision tool in regard to personality, as diagnostic tools can be used in some fields of medicine. There is no such precision tool in the field of psychiatry. We are not dealing with an organ or a system but with a human being as a totality. And he is far too complex for the state of our knowledge to pigeonhole into exact categories. The element of the unexpected and unpredictable is with us more constantly than with the average specialist.

One of the things we do know is that the entity that we call a human being is endowed with biologic energy that apparently must be discharged, and with some degree of comfort to the organism. This energy finds its outlet in the use of capacities with which the organism is endowed. Training and education may modify the method of using ability or capacity, from the muscular exercise of the aimless gestures of an infant to the highly skilled muscular exercise of a tennis player, but the fundamental fact is that energy must be expended through the use of abilities possessed. Although this has not been explained fully, it is also apparently necessary that abilities be used with some degree of feeling of power or success. This tendency toward self-realization, that is, the use of personal talents and skills with satisfaction, and the ability to reach out freely and find fulfillment with others on a realistic basis seems an important force in all of us.

One other fact that seems reasonably certain is that two major motivations underlie behavior, one biologic in origin and one social in origin. These are drives, if one may be forgiven for using the word, for satisfaction and for security. Satisfaction is derived from the release of tension in smoooth muscles. It is this simple in the beginning, but conditioning makes the process more complicated. Nevertheless the essential trigger that sets one looking for satisfaction is smooth muscle tension that is fundamentally biologic in origin. Security, on the other hand, relates to a cultural need, man being social by nature, and is a feeling of safety and certainty in relationships with other people. This security or lack of it is derived primarily from the individual's perception of himself in relation to others, as equal, inferior, superior, liked, respected, unwanted, etc. That perception and how it is handled influence profoundly the course of a person's development.

Anxiety

Anxiety, with its influence upon growth and the achievement of maturity, is a central problem in personality development. It is a strong motivation force in normal behavior and the crucial problem in emotional and behavioral disorders, for these are both an expression of and a defense against intolerable anxiety.

No one is premanently free from anxiety. A mild degree can be constructive when it provides a stimulus to action that deals directly with anxiety or removes the cause of it. It can, for example, motivate a student to do the necessary studying to pass an examination or, an even more healthy reaction, motivate her to learn something she recognizes a need to know. On the other hand, anxiety can be destructive when it either leaves the concerned individual helpless to act or overwhelms the personality. Anxiety can be aroused by external danger or by internal danger. The power to arouse anxiety from within lies in unacceptable thought, feelings, wishes, or drives which entail the loss of love or approval and the expectation of punishment. The anxiety connected with rejection and disapproval is used by adults in teaching children behavior patterns. The dangers and the potentials for healthy development are implicit in this process. How parents or parent surrogates use anxiety, how they balance it with love and affection, and to what extent they themselves are the carriers of intense anxiety are profoundly important for the developing personality. Severe and consistent disapproval by significant people is quite enough to account for lifelong severe anxiety.

Some of the source of anxiety in parents may well be related to the times in which we live. This is often, as a matter of fact, called the age of anxiety. It is a complicated world with the threat of atomic warfare close and immediate. We are in a period of rapid social change in which old and accepted values and standards of behavior have not been replaced with others of equal authority, and the result is uncertainty. At times, technical efficiency seems to be worth more than personal values. There is an increasing pressure for conformity as people become increasingly interdependent. There seems to be less use for the individual as such, with a resultant threat of a meaningless existence. Almost every one experiences insecurity in the face of the complexities of the world in which we live. However, anxiety so generated can be constructive as well as destructive. It can be used as an instrument for improvement and progress.

Raymond B. Cattell and other psychologists have been working with a new statistical technique, factor analysis, in the study of personality traits. As a result of their work, they conclude that anxiety does exist both as a state of being and as a personality trait. Anxiety is marked by a high susceptibility to annoyance, ego-weakness, guilt proneness, easy group inhibition, and rapid body tempo along with the physiologic manifestations. Two physiologic responses usually associated with anxiety, dry mouth and general muscle tension, were found to be missing in the presence of anxiety. Instead, salivary output increases and muscle tension is found primarily in the trapezius muscle. The research groups also believe, on the basis of their findings, that anxiety differs from both stress effort and neurotic adjustment. In effort stress the individual grapples with difficulties and shows strong concentration and awareness of effort. In anxiety the individual retreats and attempts escape. The researchers suggest that this may be an age of effort stress rather than an age of anxiety. It is difficult to assess the significance of such findings at the present, but the ideas do raise some interesting questions.

Organic endowment*

The newborn infant is endowed with a certain physical make-up. He is an extremely complex organism maintained by the balance of tissues, organs, and systems, their interaction with each other, and their combined interaction with their environment. Life is first of all a biochemical fact. No infant could exist without the oxygen in the atmosphere that surrounds him, any more than he could exist without lungs to absorb it, without blood to distribute it, or without tissues to utilize it. All this is organized into the unit that is "the infant."

The type of organized physical unit that the infant possesses will play a part in his personality development. Some biologic needs may be stronger than others and cause him to select from his environment certain factors to which he will respond more readily. The predominance of one type of tissue over another—ectodermal over endodermal and mesodermal —may endow him with handicaps or attributes in his search for satisfaction. His very physical appearance may have much to do with his feeling of security since practically all cultures having strong attitudes about personal appearance against which a person will be measured and found acceptable or wanting.

Suffice it to say that there is an organic matrix from which personality develops which will have a very definite influence on the direction of personality development.

Cultural influences

The kind of society into which an individual is born will unquestionably be a profound factor in the kind of personality he will develop. Character and personality take shape in a social setting. One is born with a set of potentialities for personality development, but the environment will indicate those particular traits that are to be developed and those that are to be discouraged. In fact, probably the most characteristic trait of the human being is his plasticity.

Undoubtedly the most important part of life as far as personality development is concerned is early childhood. It is within family life that the foundation for the adult personality is laid. Here basic drives or directing tendencies are modified by early interaction, and here the awareness of self is learned in relationships with others. And it is society which determines the basic pattern of family life. It is the cultural pattern into which one is born that provides and defines the behavior expectations of an individual and the roles that he must learn to fill. The system of values, the definition of behaviors that will win acceptance, and the kinds of life goals that will be important aspects of the dynamics of individual personality development are derived from the social culture.

Many kinds of behavior make more sense when this point of view is

---

*Since this textbook is written for student nurses, a review of anatomy and psysiology is omitted. Students are referred to such textbooks if review is necessary.

considered. Despite the gap between Christian theory and Christian practice, Western civilization, with its basic Christian ethic, does place a great emphasis upon the importance of the individual. Although they are changing, Eastern civilizations, on the other hand, have long placed an emphasis upon the individual not as an end in himself but as a part of something greater, the continuity of existence in which the individual is only one facet. In the light of this, even the differences in the provision of medical services between the two civilizations make sense. One is concerned with and provides for each and every individual as far as possible, whereas the other does not. On the other hand, Western civilization is accused of having succumbed to materialistic values, whereas Eastern civilizations have not. If they are true, both of these facts are probably related to the differing emphases in the cultures upon the importance of the worth of an individual life. Fortunately or unfortunately, Eastern civilizations appear to be moving, valuewise, in the direction of the West.

Although culture in specific countries or civilizations may have a considerable homogeneity, there are variations and subdivisions within them which have significance for the kind of behavior that will develop within them. Lower socioeconomic classes in the United States, for example, tend to be less disturbed by antisocial behavior than middle and upper classes. This and many other varying values leave their mark upon the personalities of people born into different classes. In addition, to complicate the understanding of behavior, the individual who is observing tends to judge behavior in terms of the social values of the class in which he grew up. As a practical point, nurses need to learn enough about the cultural backgrounds from which their patients come to use this knowledge in understanding behavior. Mexican laborers who work in the United States may not be overly impressed with our middle-class devotion to physical cleanliness, but their love of color and music have made a real contribution to American culture, especially in the Southwest. Certain ethnic groups, as part of their cultural background, learn to verbalize freely their physical complaints and pains as an accepted pattern of behavior. This needs understanding since it is almost certain to conflict with the social values of the nurse.

Actually, health behavior and attitudes in general differ in varying socioeconomic levels. The lower the social class, the less likely is the individual to seek medical help early and to utilize available health services. Also, the lower the social class, the less likely the individual is to recognize and to understand the significance of the more serious symptoms of illness.

A recent social study done by Hollingshead and Redlich in New Haven, Connecticut, indicates that social class itself is reflected by differences in types of diagnoses made and kinds of treatment given psychiatric patients. No cause-effect relationship was definitely established. One of the most disturbing facts uncovered was that patients from the upper socioeconomic classes in the community received considerably more in the way of psychotherapy, whereas patients from the lower socioeconomic classes tended to receive more organic therapy, especially electro-convulsive therapy. That value differences between high-status physicians and low-status patients were obstacles in therapy was pointed out. The need for understanding the impact of cultural patterns on behavior becomes obvious if personality development and patient behavior are to be understood.

In an epidemiologic study of psychiatric disorders done in Texas by Jaco, the concept that every individual in the population had an equal chance of becoming mentally ill did not hold true. The incidence of a first mental illness occurred more often as age increased and women had a higher incidence rate than men. In the cultural groups included in the study, the rank order was Anglo-Americans, nonwhite races, and Spanish Americans.

Infant experience

One ability the infant possesses is highly significant, the unexplained power of communication of tones of emotional feeling, or the power of empathy. He is able to sense and respond to feelings of approval or disapproval of the mother or nurse. Feelings of approval increase his sense of well-being, and the opposite feelings cause discomfort. This happens long before he is capable of understanding the meaning of either feeling or before he is capable of any discrimination in regard to experience. Although all experience is planted forever in the personality, at this time the infant has simply a vague comprehension of things as pleasant or unpleasant and a vague association of them in relation to the mother or mother-figure. Also at this period the world is simply a cosmic universe with no limitations to any single entity, either self or others. Satisfactions are achieved with the first magic tool, the cry, and comfort and discomfort are known but not understood.

Then begins the period of personal habit training with the deliberate use of approval and disapproval as tools that bend the child's behavior into approved social paths. Restraints on freedom, combined with a steady growth in the ability to differentiate perceptions, lead to the evolution of the sense of self or I, and a very important thing happens. Although not fully understood, by its very nature the organization of the individual around the self or I or ego results in an organization that henceforth seeks to perpetuate itself and maintain itself always in the direction and characteristics it acquires in its earliest stages.

What determines the direction and characteristics of the self? It comes about primarily through interaction with significant people in the environment. The use of approval or disapproval, with the resultant increase and decrease in the sense of well-being, begin to be discriminated in a crude way. The first vague grasp of cause and effect dawns, and the child, its security of paramount concern to it, begins to adapt its behavior to ensure its security. Attention becomes focused on those types of behavior which call forth some response, and other types receive no at-

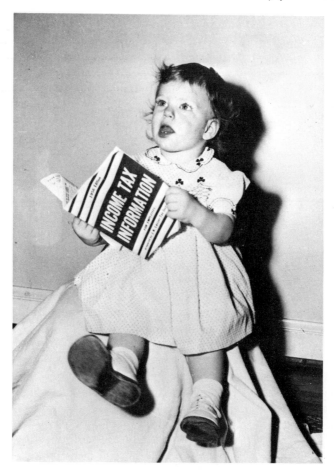

A child copies the behavior as well as the attitudes of parents.

tention since they are not significant to security. Hence, as is obvious, the more consistent the parents are, the easier will be the process of learning for the child, and less confusion and uncertainty will be built into the personality.

Several factors are of sufficient importance at this stage to merit brief discussion. The selective attention mentioned previously, that is, attention paid to *significant* things in the environment, has two results, both springing from the development of self. The experiences or parts of it which are insignificant to the child are not brought into awareness and exist only outside the awareness. These experiences are incorporated into the substratum of the self, outside of awareness. They often can, however, be integrated into the conscious self-system when attention is called to them if they do not conflict markedly with the perception or direction of the self-system. Experiences which are unpleasant, especially those which are very painful in their threat to security, are actively rejected by the self and denied access to awareness. These parts of experience, which become part of the personality, continue as dissociated parts and are not accessible to awareness. It is not that they do not have any influence on personality and behavior. They most certainly do, but without awareness of the self.

Early childhood

The child exists in an autistic world, that is, a world that has a highly personal meaning for him, not related in any way to the real world. He begins to learn to handle the ambiguous symbols of language, first investing them with his own meaning and learning as he goes to share the meaning others give them. The learning of the tool of communication with others enhances the development of self. The use of emphathy for communion with others need no longer be relied upon solely, and the newer use of language conveys approval and disapproval more accurately and easily. The process of acculturation is hastened.

The other occurrence of importance during this period is that the child adopts wholly and without question the attitudes, beliefs, and standards of those persons about him who are significant. He has not yet the experience or judgment to question them, nor can he as yet think logically to question them, although the roots of logical thinking are there in his developing ability to see cause-effect relationships. What is even more important for his future, he accepts the evaluations that others place on him without question. If he is loved and wanted, then the direction of his self will probably be strongly toward loving and wanting. If he is disliked, then the direction of his self will probably be toward hostility and dislike. If he is respected, he will probably be able to respect others. His first and most deeply learned perception of himself in relation to other people, the root of his security and his future personality development, is a reflection of how the significant persons around him perceive him.

At this moment, lest a wrong conclusion be drawn, the concept of personality as a dynamic, changing, onward moving process should be thought through again. Early experience is profoundly important for personality evolution, but it is not an absolute determinant. Corrective experience can be had at any stage of development and can often lead to a new definition of goals and a new self-perception. For example, a child who is brought up in a home in which he is unwanted and disliked will have a negative emotional attitude toward himself and others. The same child, if he is removed from his parents at school age and is *consistently* from then on respected and wanted, may and probably will change the direction of his growth toward a more positive orientation. This will not occur at once since the strength of the tendency to perpetuate the original direction of the self is strong. This explains the failure of the light-and-sweetness-you-be-kind-to-me-I'll-be-kind-to-you approach that baffles the neophyte in his first contacts with mentally ill patients. The direction of personality growth can be altered, but it will be so only through an intelligent, consistent, long-drawn-out effort. More positive aspects of the personality that exist in its dissociated part can be integrated into the self, but only slowly, because it involves a major change that will not be welcomed with open arms. Better those dangers we know than to fly to other we know not of!

Having learned to discriminate between himself and the rest of the world, the child learns that discomfort exists within himself and is not cosmic. This accompanies the development of the concept of the self or I. He now discriminates the universal experience of anxiety. This ability to feel intensely uncomfortable is both an asset and a liability. It serves as a warning or danger signal, indicating clearly that either satisfaction or security is threatened or that one threatens the other, for it is not unusual for the satisfaction of a need to threaten security.

Anxiety functions either to avoid a threat or to obscure awareness of its true significance. Here the previously determined direction of personality growth is important. A child who respects himself respects others, and his security is less often threatened. Hence his need for and use of anxiety is reduced. The child who is hostile in reaction with others brings forth many threats to his own security and hence tends to need and be dominated by anxiety more extensively.

Late childhood

Having absorbed and accepted the standards, codes, attitudes, and evaluation of himself of the significant persons in his infancy and childhood, the growing child shows a new capacity that his biologic endowment of energy forces him to use. This capacity is the continuing necessity to expand his activities, to reach out, and to interact with widening circles. He needs more companionship of his own age and group and seeks it. If playmates do not exist, he creates them in phantasy. Now he learns cooperation, accomplishing things with other personalities. If his attitude toward himself is sound, his progress will be rapid, and his sense of well-being will be enhanced. So in a steady forward direction, the child is fitted to his culture, and his culture is fitted to him.

The association with other children in play activity is a vital learning experience. The child has already developed social skills of one degree or another, patterns and ways of interacting with others which are designed to meet his needs and promote his security. In play with others he learns new roles, more independent ones. He learns a wider range of roles and develops a greater capacity for give and take. His sense of belonging widens. Old techniques that are unsuccessful in the new milieu may be discarded for better ones or may be reserved for use only in the home situation where they may continue to be effective. However, even in the home situation there is ordinarily steady pressure toward the use of more mature techniques in social relationships and toward the curbing of immediate satisfactions in the interests of the greater satisfactions of delayed pleasures and the satisfactions of others. If the child is relatively secure, he learns and progresses, exploring with both failure and success, and defines

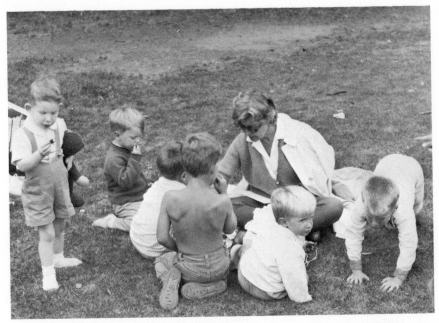

Play activities are an essential element in the social development of children.

for himself a status and prestige on ever-widening horizons that are acceptable to himself and to the other persons with whom he establishes relationships. He interchanges roles as necessary with increasing flexibility and ease. If, however, he is insecure, the road is apt to be rocky.

Adolescence

Culture places one more period of crisis on the way toward adulthood and that is the period of adolescence. The maturing of the sexual drive at this period is accompanied by considerable emotional stress and reorientation of goals in terms of sexual objectives. How much of the emotional stress is biologic in origin and how much culturally induced is a moot point. There exist societies in which adolescence represents no struggle. Here the adjustment will be largely determined by the previous pattern since it will be modeled on past experiences which tend to prevent radical newness in interpersonal situations. The significance of adolescence lies in the fact that it represents a crisis period, and the destructive and constructive potentialities are somewhat greater than average.

Adolescence is a period rife with conflicts. The drive toward independence is coupled with comparatively immature judgment which makes it a risk. The desire for independence usually draws conscious or unconscious resistance from the parents. The strong need to be exactly like one's peers opposes parental demands. The sensitive need for complete approval is endangered by the uneven physical development that is accompanied by awkwardness and physical peculiarities of appearance. The standards of one's own generation appear so much more modern and worthwhile than the standards of parents, so that family identification becomes a little painful. This phenomenon challenges parents and may produce changes in parent-child relationships. There is a need and wish both to be alone and develop one's own set of values and to be with others and share their values. There is usually a desire for adult privileges and an apprehension about adult responsibilities. There is a physical readiness for sexual maturity and a cultural block in the way of its achievement. On the whole, adolescence is a period of ambivalence. The secure child can survive it, pass through it, and emerge from it an adult. The insecure child will, of course, find it more painful although he too may eventually emerge an adult in more than a physical sense.

Maturity

The ultimate goal of healthy personality development is an adult capable of predominantly positive emotional orientation toward others, of initiative, and of responsibility. The final goal is achieved when the individual is capable of accepting the satisfaction and security of another as being of equal importance with his own. He is then capable of mature, adult love.

There exists within all of us a strong tendency to achieve mental health. Most persons seek experience which corrects deficiencies in acculturation. Sometimes this is with good results and sometimes it is disastrous. One rebelliously defiant young student nurse was discovered to be a person with a deep abiding resentment of female authority which grew out of personal experience with her domineering mother. In all her choices of vocation, there are few occupations in which she could have come more quickly to grips with her basic problems than in the nursing field where female authority, truly authoritarian in nature, is all too often the accepted pattern. Unfortunately, the student failed to resolve her conflicts and finally forced her own removal from the school of nursing. Such experiences are not always so unfortunate, especially if positive attitudes exist within the self as resources.

The point to keep always in mind is that the personality, conscious and unconscious, is never fixed, but always fluid and therefore capable of change. And since the basic orientation is forward and toward health, however devious the present path, no person is ever hopeless.

Developmental stages

"In the process of reaching psychosocial maturity, as pointed out by Erikson, every person goes through certain developmental stages, each featured by a developmental task that must be successfully completed if the succeeding tasks are to be resolved in turn. Although any given developmental task may be successfully completed at its appropriate stage, it is never completed for all time, since regression may occur, or stress may arouse again an interplay between the positive and the negative outcomes inherent in the task.

"During the period of infancy one of the major tasks confronting the new individual is the development of trust—trust in one's self, in the environment and the people in it, and in the meaningfulness of existence. Such a sense of trust is derived through the close and intimate association with mother or mother surrogate. A continuous and consistent warm and supportive relationship results in a basic and essential sense of trust. The sense of trust rests on a feeling of inner goodness that is an outgrowth of the relationship. A mother-infant relationship that is inconsistent, cold, or rejecting, or that provides little or sporadic support provides experience that builds mistrust into the basic personality of the infant. The relationship is most sensitive at the period when the child experiences a sense of loss as he discriminates himself from his environment and recognizes his mother as a separate entity. The inability to trust the self and its environment can cripple personality development and deprive the growing individual of those interpersonal relationships and experiences which are essential to growth and self-realization.

"The second developmental stage occurs in early childhood, and the developmental task at this age is the establishment of a sense of autonomy. It is a result of the need to establish a differentiation between the self and its own will and the pressures of outside influences. It begins with the period of 'I,' 'We,' and 'No,' being a period of concern with self and with resistance to outside pressures. The favorable outcome of this crisis is a development of a sense of autonomy on the part of the growing child. The negative outcome is a sense of doubt and shame, usually the result of a consistent loss in the battle of 'No's' with people who are bigger and stronger.

"The third developmental stage is the play age, and the developmental task is the establishment of initiative. The freedom to explore and to reach security in taking the initiative in action comes as the child moves out of the home and family and into his immediate community. The curiosity and the exploration and the accompanying fantasies can also lead to feelings of guilt with its resulting anxiety. If the guilt is reinforced rather than the curiosity, exploration and initiative in action, the negative outcome of guilt may result, and the growing personality may develop a sense of 'badness,' with restrictions in his initiative in later stages of development. This is also the period of the development of conscience.

"The next developmental stage is the school age, and the growing personality confronts the task of developing the trait of industry which is essential for the capacity to enjoy work. In this stage, the world expands again, and the skills and tools in working and relating to the world are developed. The child learns to work with others and to produce things, both individually and with others. It is important for the growing personality that the initiative in action developed in the preceding stage amount to something—that what results reflects competence and worth. The dan-

ger in this period is the development of a sense of inferiority and medioc-
rity, usually a result of lack of recognition for efforts.

"The fifth developmental stage occurs in puberty and adolescence, and
the developmental task is the achievement of a sense of identity. Rapid
physical development and the advent of sexual maturity precipitate the
crisis of concentration or diffusion—the sense of one's own identity or diffusion of identity that results from attempting to be too many things to
too many persons. The dangers of this period are either diffusion of identity
or a negative identity, an attempt to become what others do not want the
adolescent to become.

"The sixth developmental stage is young adulthood, and the developmental task is the ability to establish intimate relationships with others.
The negative alternate choice is isolation. Having established a sense of
his own identity and some degree of harmony within himself, the young
adult becomes capable of investing some of himself in others. This means
the establishment of friendships and eventually a satisfying and satisfactory marriage. If close relationships with others threatens a weak sense
of self identity, isolation ensues and restricts individual ability to achieve
self-realization.

"The seventh developmental stage is adulthood, in which the developmental task is generativity, and the negative resolution is self-absorption.
Generativity is reflected in the individual's establishment and guiding of
the next generation. Self-absorption is again a restricted factor in self-realization and results in a sense of stagnation.

"The last developmental stage, and the last adult crisis, comes in the
late middle or late years of life in which man sums up his personal balance. The result is either a sense of integrity or a sense of despair and disgust. Integrity is achieved when the individual accepts responsibility for
what his life has been and finds it has both internal and external worth."[*]

---

[*]From Matheney, Ruth V.: Nolan, Breda T., Ehrhart, Alice M., Griffin, Gerald J., and
Griffin, Joanne King: Fundamentals of patient-centered nursing, St. Louis, 1964, The
C. V. Mosby Co., pp. 62-63.

References

Cameron, Norman: The psychology of behavior disorders, New York, 1947, Houghton
   Mifflin Co., pp. 15-52.
Cattell, Raymond B.: The nature and measurement of anxiety, Scientific American
   208:96-104, Mar. 1963.
Erikson, Erik H.: Childhood in society, New York, 1950, W. W. Norton & Co., pp.
   219-234.
Fromm-Reichmann, Frieda: Psychiatric aspects of anxiety, In Stein, M., Vidich, A. J.,
   and White, D. M., editors: Identity and anxiety, Glencoe, Ill., 1960, Free Press, pp.
   129-141.
Hollingshead, August B., and Redlich, Frederick C.: Social class and mental illness,
   New York, 1958, John Wiley & Sons, Inc., p. 442.
Jaco, E. Gartly: The social epidemiology of mental disorders, New York, 1960, Russell
   Sage Foundation.

Kariel, Patricia E.: The dynamics of behavior in relation to health, Nursing Outlook **10**:402-405, June 1962.

May, Rollo: Centrality of the problem of anxiety in our day. In Stein, M., Vidich, A. J., and White, D. M., editors: Identity and anxiety, Glenco, Ill., 1960, Free Press, pp. 120-128.

Mullahy, Patrick, editor: A study of interpersonal relationships, New York, 1949, Hermitage House, Inc.

Neylan, Margaret Prowse: Anxiety, American Journal of Nursing **62**:110-111, May 1962.

Peplau, Hildegarde E.: Interpersonal relations in nursing, New York, 1952. G. P. Putnam's Sons, pp. 161-259.

Sullivan, Harry Stack: Conceptions of modern psychiatry, Washington, D. C., 1947. William Alanson White Psychiatric Foundation, pp. 1-42, 119-147.

Chapter iv

Psychoanalytic theory
of personality development

Varying schools of thought or disciplines exist in the field of psychiatry. Although the general trend in America has been eclectic in nature, many schools with varying interpretations of personality development do exist. Among the more important are the schools of psychoanalytic thought, all based upon the orthodox views originating with Sigmund Freud. Since psychoanalysis has been profoundly important historically, a brief outline of its major points of view and contributions will be included here. Sigmund Freud revolutionized the thinking of the profession about mental illness, about personality development, and about the treatment of personality deviations. All psychiatric thinking today rests on the ground work of his insights into human behavior.

Structure of personality

The structure of personality, according to Freud, consists of three basic parts whose internal conflict and maintenance of balance are the factors that produce what we call behavior. These three components of personality are the id, the ego, and the superego. Concerned only with striving after pleasure and satisfaction, the id is the raw stuff of personality, the primitive and biologic drives and urges. It is also the reservoir of psychic energy, called the libido by the analysts. The id is that part of the personality with which we are born, a personality ruled only by the pleasure principle. Chronologically, the ego is developed next and arises from the experience of frustration or thwarting of immediate satisfaction. It is the part of the self most closely in touch with reality and is roughly equivalent to what is meant by self or conscious awareness. The ego develops to mediate between the strivings of the id and the demands of the environment so that satisfactions may be achieved in a manner which coincides with physical and social reality. As the ego develops, the reality principle supercedes or operates in concert with the pleasure principle in guiding behavior. The relative strength of each will be determined by the comparative

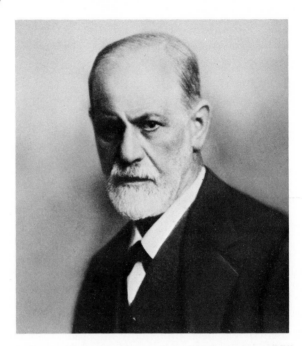

Sigmund Freud, the founder of the psychoanalytic movement.
(Courtesy Bettman Archive, Inc.)

strength of the id and the ego in the total personality. The superego develops later than the other two aspects of personality and represents the acceptance of the responsibility for the regulation of his own conduct by the individual. The superego is roughly equivalent to conscience, or the sense of right and wrong. Its beginning occurs primarily by acceptance early in life of the standards of the persons who are most important to the child, and it is first evidence when the child feels within himself that his behavior is right or wrong.

The id then is primarily biologic in nature and biologically conditioned. It is the id which says, "I want." The ego is derived from physical reality and says, "Better not because you will get hurt." The superego is social or cultural in origin and says, "You can't do that because it is wrong." There is, of course, constant conflict between the id and the superego and potential conflict between any two of them. From these conflicts comes the sources of behavior, and the resolution of conflicts is in the direction of growth. Without conflict and frustration, there would be no growth.

Topography of the self

Conflicts do not always occur in the individual's awareness. One of Freud's greatest contributions to an understanding of human behavior was his popularization of the concept of the unconscious. Not all mental activity, in fact only a small part of it, is conscious. The mind consists roughly of three overlapping divisions: the conscious, the subconscious, and the unconscious. By the conscious is meant that part of the mind which is immediately focused in awareness. The subconscious is that part which can be recalled and brought to awareness at will. The unconscious is the reservoir of memories, experiences, and emotions which cannot be recalled. This part is by far the largest part of mental activity and is proportionately equivalent to the submerged part of an iceberg. Parts of the id, ego, and superego exist in all strata of the conscious and the unconscious; although the larger part of the id is in the unconscious.

Mental mechanisms

Behavior occurs because of conflict between or among the id, ego, and superego which may be wholly conscious or wholly unconscious, or any combination thereof. The economic aspect of behavior lies in the fact that it resolves conflict. The method may be unhealthy and lead to further conflict. Nonetheless, conflict situations are resolved with the least possible expenditure of energy. The method of resolution is through the use of certain methods of thinking, or mental mechanisms, which eliminate conflict or reduce its severity. Since these mechanisms are important to an understanding of the significance of behavior, the most important will be identified. They are not wholly clear-cut. On the contrary, they often overlap and may so often be used in conjunction with each other that in actual behavior it may be almost impossible to identify them exclusively.

Denial, plain ordinary rejection, is a method of resolving conflict that all persons use to some extent. We simply refuse to face facts as they are. A man is not a coward to himself, no matter how cowardly his behavior. He may go further and reinforce the denial, but it is often the only step taken. A thing is just not so if it produces pain or conflict for it to be that way. In fact, the denial of illness is a fairly common behavior pattern on medical and surgical patient care units. The rejection of physical illness can have serious consequences for a patient with a major health problem.

Repression is a more complicated mechanism in which unpleasant or unacceptable experiences, emotions, or motivations are actively forced into the unconscious and kept there. The emotional context of repressed material may be a powerful source of motivation for behavior, but the individual is never aware of the true source or association of the emotion. A child frustrated and downtrodden by a severe parent may spend his life as a rebel against authority, always thinking he is activated by altruistic motives, yet always acting out his conflict with his parent. He is quite firmly sure that he loves and has always loved that particular parent. Repression operates wholly on an unconscious level.

Conversion is exactly what it says—strong emotional conflicts are expresed as or converted into physical symptoms. The boy who hates his father and is torn between the desire to strike him and fear of the consequences if he does so develops a paralyzed arm. The conflict is resolved. He cannot strike his father even if he wishes to, and the situation carries no threat of retaliation. In addition, the boy secures sympathy and attention for his symptom. The mechanism of conversion also operates wholly on an unconscious level. Interestingly, the utilization of the mental mechanism of conversion is strongly influenced by cultural factors. A better educated public now uses the mechanism more subtly than used to be true in the past.

Regression is a retreat from the present pattern to past levels of behavior. It occurs when discomfort becomes intense, and the individual returns to previous patterns of behavior that were successful in earlier stages of development. All people use this mechanism sometimes, usually under temporary stress when they resort to childish methods to obtain their goals. Tears and temper tantrums in adults are sometimes very effective, even though they may not be adult forms of behavior. Actually, some degree of regression frequently accompanies the occurrence of physical illness, and regressed behavior of varying degrees of intensity is found in most patients in general hospitals. Regression is a mechanism exhibited to an extreme degree by mentally ill patients who may retreat all the way back to the infantile level. Its ultimate illustration is the severely ill patient who curls into fetal position and remains there obstinately.

Sublimation is a rather constructive method of resolving conflict if it is successful. The mechanism consists of using the energy involved in a primitive impulse, not acceptable in its frank and direct expression, in an activity that is socially constructive. A man who has strong sexual drives and utilizes that energy in writing poetry or painting nude women, doing it well, and thereby contributing to the arts is an excellent example.

Reaction formation or overcompensation is an interesting mechanism. It is a means for disguising from the self the possession of an unacceptable desire or drive by developing its exact opposite to an extreme degree. It often, however, reveals its nature to the alert observer by the many slips made and the degree of extremity of the trait which seems uncalled for. The person who is excessively sweet and polite under any and all circumstances is often a very hostile person who finds it necessary to disguise her hostility from herself and others. She usually makes others uncomfortable in the process, which hints at the underlying hostility. An interesting illustration of reaction formation is to be found in letters to the editor from some public-spirited citizens who are opposed to the vivisection of animals in the study of disease. Such letters, with their description in cruel and bloody detail of what ought to happen to the persons involved, reveal their writers' basic hostility.

Rationalization is the joy and delight of the average human being. It is simply finding a logical reason for the things one wants to do and is self-deception at its subtle best. The woman who buys a dress she could well do without and cannot really afford, but who can explain its purchase satisfactorily to her husband and herself, is a good example. The self-deception is in regard to the real motivation for behavior.

Identification is a very important mechanism in the process of adjusting to culture. Closely related to it is the mechanism of introjection, and since the difference in the two seems to be mainly one of degree, their definitions may be considered together. The basic process in both mechanisms is the acceptance of persons, ideas, or ideals outside the self, feeling with them as though they were part of the self, and finally integrating them into the core of one's own personality. If there is a difference between identification and introjection, identification would include the first two elements in the definition, and the addition of the third would make the mechanism introjection. The acceptance of the standards of parents and molding behavior to meet those standards on one's own initiative is both identification and introjection. The parents have been identified with, and their standards have been introjected.

Projection is a very popular method of resolving conflicts and one that dominates the behavior of certain types of personalities. Projection is the perception of thinking, feeling, or motor activity as having its origin outside the self when in reality its origin is in the personality of the perceiver. Its purpose is obviously self-protective since that which is unacceptable to the self can be projected on the environment, and self-esteem can thereby be maintained. For example, as a simple illustration, who was ever wrong in a heated argument? The other fellow, of course. In the severely mentally ill patient, auditory hallucinations can and do occur, that is, the patient hears voices when there are no voices to hear. The only source for such voices is in the thoughts of the patient himself which, being too unpleasant to tolerate as coming from the self, are perceived as coming from the environment. This is wholly uncontrolled projection which is a danger signal. Actually, strange as such behavior may seem, it is not different in nature or process from the common projection that operates when we place the blame for our difficulties on others. We project faults or failures that are our own. When grades are low, it is the teacher's fault; when the boss loses his temper at a mistake, it is because of his nasty disposition. Used too extensively, the mechanism of projection can grow to dominate behavior and lead to serious maladjustment.

Displacement is the transference of emotion from one object, situation, or idea to another. Being angry with one's wife and kicking the dog, missing a shot and breaking the golf club, and being angry at the charge nurse and snapping at a patient are all examples of displacement.

Transference is in a sense a form of displacement, except that its meaning is more restricted. It means the shifting of feelings of strong positive or negative emotional attachment from one object or person to another. If the feeling is love, we speak of a positive transference and if hate, of a negative transference. Transference forms the basis for most therapeutic relationships.

Symbolization, without the use of which none of us could ever adapt to our culture, means that one idea or object stands for another. The distinction between a symbol and the thing symbolized and how they stand for and represent each other is one of the most confusing lessons a child must master. Many mentally ill patients appear to be in exactly this state of confusion. WORD is only four printed letters, but it means one of the tools of language. A single gesture can symbolize or hold the entire meaning of loved person. Symbols have both general and personal meaning. This must be remembered since symbolization is used extensively in organizing experience within the personality, and the method of using symbols is one key to the personality.

Personality development

The Freudian psychoanalytic school equates personality development with psychosexual development. Freud advanced the very unpopular theory that the sexual instinct does not spring into being suddenly and completely mature at adolescence. Rather he held that its appearance at this period was the culmination of all the stages through which the individual had passed. Sex is interpreted more broadly than it tends to be in our culture, in which the meaning of the word is restricted to genital activity. Freud saw the maturation of the sex instinct as the last step in the maturation of emotional development. Therefore, personality development is explained through its core or center, which is psychosexual development.

The actual process of birth, the individual's first traumatic experience, does have psychologic significance, but its depth and extent are not clearly defined. The newborn child is a helpless person, largely id, and primarily physiologic in expression. Feeding at the breast is his most important activity and source of greatest pleasure. Tension relief is achieved by sucking or swallowing, and there seems to be a sucking need that is independent of hunger satisfaction. For that reason, the earliest stage of development is called the oral sucking stage. The child is a passive dependent person, ruled completely by the pleasure principle. He derives satisfaction that is autoerotic in nature, that is, he experiences pleasure without any knowledge of self and hence no self-love. The oral sucking stage is brought to an end by the frustration involved in weaning which produces the first major trauma and the first major conflict.

By the process of weaning, the child is forced to develop a more differentiated personality to cope with his conflict. He begins to recognize reality and its demands and to develop ideas of himself as an individual. His ego begins to emerge, and he shows evidences of narcissism or self-love. He cuts teeth and now has the equipment to exhibit aggressiveness. The conflict over the frustration of weaning is resolved through the development of oral aggressive behavior. Pleasure is found in biting, as well as in sucking. At this time the infant shows ambivalence toward his mother—she is both a source of pleasure, in feeding and physical comfort, and a source of dissatisfaction because of the weaning process. Also at this time come further demands for conformity in the beginning of training in habits of personal cleanliness. The final weaning, the training in cleanliness, and the possible appearance of another child combine to produce the second major traumatic experience. The resolution of this conflict results in strengthening of the ego and development of the reality principle as a factor in the motivation of behavior although the pleasure principle continues its domination. This period of development, the oral aggressive, overlaps markedly the stage which succeeds it, the anal expulsive stage.

The child learns early to enjoy the release of tension that accompanies the evacuation of the bowels and the bladder. He also comes to learn that the parents place tremendous importance on urine and feces being deposited at specific places and times. He learns to look on urine and feces as being something dirty on one hand and as something valuable to be retained on the other hand. Since the ego and the sense of reality become well developed during this period, the child achieves a sense of power through control of evacuation. Not only are urine and feces a means of securing rewards and affection, but they are also amenable to being used for aggressive purposes. The child reaches the stage at which he goes through a phase of reality testing. He perceives the consequences of giving in to the pleasure principle under certain circumstances. If the course of development has been relatively normal, from here on pleasurable acts will be generally carried out with a certain respect for reality and the probable consequences of the act. Two effects of the toilet training period are, first, development of the anal retentive period and, second, the vague beginnings of the superego or conscience. The child realizes the social value of retaining, controlling, and possessing feces. In addition, all excreta have an independent value for him. On the one hand, they are valuable as gifts to please the parents, but under certain conditions they are dirty and may be insults. Some of this childhood confusion may well continue throughout life. The final frustration of the anal period occurs about the end of the fourth year when the child must finally give up the pleasures of the particular period. At the same time, reality has taught him that he is an individual, and, worse yet, it now dawns on him that he is not the most important individual in existence or even in his own family. In fact, he realizes dimly that his parents may even be more important to each other than he is to either of them. This is a blow. The realization of his relative unimportance is the conflict that precipitates the phallic period.

Children by this time are aware of the physical differences between the sexes and exhibit curiosity about it. The chief source of pleasure is deflected from the anal to the genital region. Masturbation is a common experience. This is primarily narcissistic in character—the child is interested in himself and his own genitalia. There exists considerable confusion in the mind of the child about the use of sexual organs, and he begins to have ideas about sexuality. For the first time comes a sense of a need for others as an object of sexual activity, and the choice naturally falls upon the parents. They are closer to the child emotionally than anyone else, and they represent power and prestige. Knowing the difference between sexes, the child wonders why in rather concrete terms. It occurs to the boy that loss of the penis is possible and to the girl that she has lost hers. This situation in the male leads to the Oedipus situation, the castration complex, and ultimately to the repression of infantile sexuality.

The male child was first dependent on his mother, and it is natural when he develops the first ideas of sexuality that he chooses his mother as a love object. He also realizes that his mother belongs to his father and that the latter is a formidable rival. He realizes that there are serious consequences if he should become a real rival for his mother's affections, and connecting the penis vaguely with the sexual act, he fears its loss. This fear of castration leads to a repression of infantile sexuality since any sexual expression of his perference for his mother is dangerous. However, since the child loves both parents, he resolves the conflict by identifying with the father and introjecting his standards. This further strengthens the superego, whose appearance was begun during the anal stage of development, through complete acceptance as one's own of the attributes and standards of the parent. Such a solution, ending with identification with the parent of the same sex, is a positive resolution and a normal course of events. The resulting repression of all infantile sexuality brings the child to the latency period.

The Electra complex in the female follows a slightly different sequence of events. Her first love object, during the oral and anal stages, is the mother. A growing awareness of sexuality during the phallic stage of development causes her to choose her father as her love object, and the mother is seen as the rival for his affections. Since the penis is already lost, she has less immediate fear and goes through the conflicts of this period more slowly than a boy. Finally, however, she may begin to see the possibility of having a child as a compensation for the loss of the penis and may then identify with the mother, whose voice becomes her superego.

Both the male and female may go through the Oedipus situation in a negative fashion and identify with the wrong parent or with neither. A successful resolution of the Oedipal situation is essential to healthy personality development.

Once infantile sexuality is repressed, the child is not consciously concerned with sexual matters. All such urges are sublimated in education and play. The child spends this time learning how to behave in society.

At the age of puberty, there is a gradual revival of all the infantile sexual stages. The revival of the phallic period dominates, but the phallic interest gradually develops into real genital interests. Oral and anal interests also occur and bathroom humor is popular. Since the threat of castration is not wholly gone and narcissism still very evident, the first object in this stage is usually of the same sex, the normal homosexual period. Interest turns gradually and tentatively to the other sex. The first love affair is usually phallic since, in finding himself as an adult, the individual is concerned primarily with himself as a lover. The final genital stage, true heterosexuality, is reached when the individual is concerned primarily with the love object.

It should be clearly understood that the stages of development shade and merge into successive stages and that interests of each stage persist as permanent parts of the personality. Each stage has its particular frustration and major trauma, and successful resolution of the conflict of each is essential to normal development. The unresolved conflict remains in the unconscious and from there motivates behavior in an unhealthy fashion and in unhealthy directions.

Contributions since Freud

Some of Freud's own pupils and later students of behavior who followed in his path have differed with his theories and have introduced new concepts in the field of psychoanalytic thought. A few of the more important deviations from Freud's theories are described very briefly in the following paragraphs.

Alfred Adler, a follower of Freud in the early psychoanalytic move-

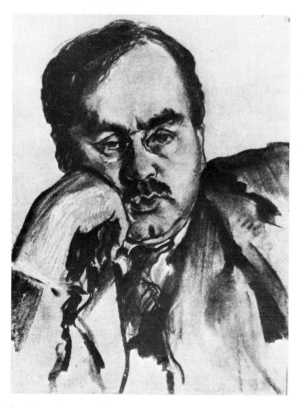

Alfred Adler, the founder of the school of individual psychology.
(Courtesy Bettman Archive, Inc.)

ment, broke with the master and founded an independent school known as individual psychology. One of the major tenets of Freud that he discarded was the libido theory based upon the importance of infantile sexuality. He turned toward the area of interpersonal interactions, particularly attitudes toward the self and others, as a basis for a theory of personality development. Beginning with the helplessness of the infant as a primary and influential experience, he conceived personality as beginning from a feeling of inferiority and striving throughout life toward superiority, power, mastery, and perfection. Organic inferiority, or congenital body defect or weakness, determined the areas in which superiority was sought or struggle avoided. The organic inferiority itself was not considered as significant as the individual's and other's attitude toward it. (Adler certainly popularized the expression "inferiority complex" in the American language.) Adler interpreted social feeling and interest, courage, and common sense (reality testing) as the usual attributes of normal human beings. He also supported the thesis that all behavior is goal directed; the specific personal goal of the individual and his methods of trying to achieve that goal constituted the individual's "life style." Change in a life style that has resulted in maladaptation could be accomplished by changing the life goal. Adler also emphasized two currently popular concepts: the psychologic unity of man and man's genuine human potential.

Carl Jung, who also was active in the early psychoanalytic movement, also differed from Freud on some basic tenets, and as a result started his own school known as analytical psychology. He interpreted the libido as a single life energy with many aspects and expressions and with less emphasis upon the *central* importance of sexual development for personality growth. The libido tends to follow one of two basic attitudes: introversion, subjective and inner directed, and extroversion, objective and outward directed. Both attitudes are necessary for a full and rich life, and the extreme or one-sided development of one attitude results in an unconscious development of the other where the second attitude can, from the unconscious, lead to conflict and maladaptation. Jung also identified four functions of personality—sensation, intuition, feeling, and thinking—and thought that behavior could be explained in terms of the balance of attitudes and functions that characterize the mode of operation of any given individual. Sensation and intuition are modes of apprehension of the world, sensation representing concern with the here and now and intuition representing concern with what things have been or will be. Feeling and thinking are judgmental in nature, with feeling being concerned with a sense of values and thinking with what things are in abstract. Again, all functions in balance are necessary for healthy living, and the overdevelopment of any one function results in the unconscious overdevelopment of its opposite, with a consequent threat to mental health. In studying patients, Jung emphasized a distinction between image and symbol; the former is a sign that represents agreed upon concepts (that is, the flag), and a symbol represents a deep personal individual dream or vision. The

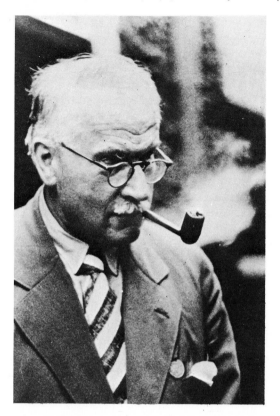

Carl Jung, the founder of the school of analytic psychology.
(Courtesy Bettman Archive, Inc.)

cross, for example, could be a sign to one person and a symbol to another, depending upon its personal meaning. One of the important sources of symbols is the collective unconscious, the sum of the experiences of the human race, which is found in the deep unconscious. Jung felt that his analytic school was more firmly rooted in the present and the future than Freud's school of thought.

Otto Rank was another of the early psychoanalysts who broke with Freudian psychology on some aspects of basic concepts. Rank was impressed with the significance of the birth trauma for personality development and considered it a primary factor. A major human goal is return to the womb, and a major human terror is separation. The anxiety produced by separation is a universal experience, and this primal anxiety is suppressed. Rank emphasized the personality-as-a-whole and the "will" of the individual, the will being the integrative factor or the *active* relationship of the person to himself and his world. The will develops as a counter-will toward others in the process of learning to distinguish one's self as an individual, separate from others. This rebellion or differentiation arouses guilt, and it is the successful resolution of such guilt that represents both the healthy person and the goal of therapy. The ultimate goal is both separation and union, learning to accept one's own will and the will of others while belonging and caring for others. Rank's views have had more impact on the applied social sciences than upon medicine.

Karen Horney has also had considerable influence within the psychoanalytic movement, and she has developed a school of thought that utilizes the process of adaptation to life situations as an explanation for personality development. She attributes to man the inherent desire and ability to change, to grow, and to expand, not merely to avoid pain or suffering. A prime motivating factor in behavior is the need for security, which is not a universal factor but one that operates when security is threatened. She believes that the infant's sense of helplessness leads not to a drive for mastery or power since, with his potential, the infant need not always feel helpless. However, she does consider that the infant's feelings of helplessness, when it does occur, leads to an exaggerated need for security and forms the background for a neurotic adjustment. The social orientation of Horney's concepts are evidenced by her belief that one of man's basic needs is to value himself and to be valued by others. She also believes that the individual develops an ideal self-image which constitutes an integrating factor in behavior. Horney also treats conflict as essentially pathogenic, with a neurotic reaction involving repression of part of the conflict. The repressed material in the unconscious continues to influence behavior to a great extent. Horney, like others, also emphasizes the unity of man and his functioning as a total person.

The name of Harry Stack Sullivan is associated with the so-called interpersonal school of the William Alanson White Psychiatric Foundation. According to his point of view, the crucial aspects of personality development are to be found in personal interrelationships. The first great human need is for a reduction of biologic tension, but the infant soon becomes aware of the relationship of the feelings of others toward him and the existence of inward tensions. He begins to adjust his behavior accordingly, and the need for security assumes increasing importance as a motivating factor in behavior. The factors of tension reduction and security need combine to become the major behavior goals of any given individual. Such goals require a feeling of approval and prestige to avoid the production of anxiety. The individual's self-concept, self-image or "self-dynamism" organizes behavior, and the self-concept is built into the individual as a result of his experiences with significant other persons in his environment. It is built to a great extent on the reflected appraisals of significant others. Sullivan thus emphasizes social factors as extremely significant for personality development, especially interpersonal relationships and the self-concept in relation to them.

Erich Fromm, too, has focused upon the healthy potential for growth and self-realization of man as a central idea in personality development, but he has given this concept a somewhat different emphasis. Man represents the highest order of animal, and one of his most human character-istics is relative freedom from internal and external influences. Man has moved increasingly toward the independent use of rational choice, and it is this historic evolution that is a basic factor in personality development. The major need of a human being is to find meaning in life through the use of his own powers. The basic human conflict lies between the security given by following instincts or rigid social mores and the use of reasoned solutions to the problems of existence. For Fromm, new solutions produce new problems, requiring new solutions. It is this progressive movement toward rational living that constitutes growth and development. Since man's experience is basically social, his satisfactions are socially oriented. Fulfillment and the meaning of life are derived from productive work and the loving relationship with others.

Regardless of the specific school, all psychoanalytic groups agree upon at least four basic concepts:

1. Behavior has meaning and is not determined by chance.
2. The unconscious plays an active role in determining behavior.
3. All behavior is goal directed.
4. The early years of life are extremely important for personality development.

Needless to say, the acceptance of the four basic concepts is not restricted to psychoanalytic thinking.

In general, the new concepts added to psychoanalysis by those who followed Freud have tended to broaden the basis of personality development beyond a strictly psychosexual one, have introduced a greater emphasis upon social and cultural factors in personality development, and have placed a greater emphasis upon the drive within the individual to seek health.

References

Brill, A. A.: Freud's contribution to psychiatry, New York, 1944, W. W. Norton & Co., Inc.

Brill, A. A.: The basic writings of Sigmund Freud, New York, 1938, Modern Library, Inc.

Committee on Psychiatric Nursing, N.L.N.E.: Psychological concepts of personality development, American Journal of Nursing **50**:122-125, Feb. 1950; **50**:182-184, Mar. 1950; **50**:242-243, April 1950.

Freud, Sigmund: A general introduction to psychoanalysis, Garden City, N. Y., 1943, Garden City Publishing Co.

Munroe, Ruth L: Schools of psychoanalytic thought, New York, 1955, The Dryden Press, Inc.

Thompson, Clara: The different schools of psychoanalysis, American Journal of Nursing **57**:1304-1307, Oct. 1957.

Chapter 7

Deviate patterns
of behavior

F

Definition of deviate patterns

rom the previous discussion of personality development, it becomes apparent that there are numerous opportunities for the individual to acquire handicaps that will interfere with his ability to adjust to life. Organic lack or destruction, traumatic experience, or the acquisition of unhealthy attitudes may lead to a pattern of behavior that seriously hampers the attainment of satisfactions or security in a manner that is acceptable to the person or to the society in which he lives. When this occurs, the degree of personality impairment is a measure of the state of mental health.

For practical purposes, mental health may be defined as the abilities to develop a realistic and accepting self-knowledge, to feel genuine concern for others, to be more inner-directed than outer-directed, to take care of the self without hurting others in the process, and to tolerate stress and frustrations. Such abilities are determined largely by the individual's perception of himself in relation to others, being dependent upon original endowment and past experience. The degree of mental health of any given person fluctuates from day to day and from situation to situation; yet it tends to have a certain continuity and consistency. There is a wide range of degrees of mental health that shade so subtly into each other that hard and fast lines to distinguish between its presence or absence are all but impossible. In addition, the final judgment as to the existence of mental illness itself is cultural in nature, and certain types of maladjustment are more socially acceptable than others. Types of behavior that are bizarre, strange, or queer or that violate cultural standards that have a strong emotional impact are usually labelled as symptoms of mental illness, and society feels impelled to take action in regard to such conduct. Other types of behavior which may also indicate a lack of mental health may be ignored or accepted. For example, a person who is withdrawn and avoids relationships with others may well be regarded as a little queer but is seldom recognized as being as sick as he is. On the other hand, a person who violates sexual standards flagrantly, perhaps by exposing himself in public, calls for prompt attention. One is quickly categorized as mentally ill; the other has to prove it.

The violation of social customs, especially in sensitive areas, draws from society a punitive reaction. The Joint Commission on Mental Illness and Mental Health pointed out the significance of this fact for the mentally ill patient and for the quality of the care he receives. The mentally ill patient does not appeal to the sympathy of the public as does the physically ill patient. Instead, the type of symptoms presented by the mentally ill are in areas of behavior that have resulted in public rejection.

The point of origin of behavior deviations lies in the motivations that are acquired through experience. Behavior is seldom frankly psychotic as an objective phenomenon—it is behavior as seen in the total situation, its appropriateness and its effectiveness in contributing to security, that is important. A man thoroughly frightened and racing wildly down the street screaming for help is not in the least maladjusted if there happens to be a man-eating tiger at his heels; quite the reverse is true if the flight was precipitated by some vague feeling of anxiety that had no obvious objective stimulus.

Anxiety, that intense sense of personal discomfort, is a profound motivator of behavior. It occurs when the self-esteem of an individual is threatened, from the outside or inside. The situations that call it forth are usually the result of past experience. Some of us are made anxious by love, some by hate, and some by indifference. The method of resolving the conflict produced and reducing the anxiety is largely that of previous patterns of behavior. The elements of newness or uniqueness in any situation may bring about a change in the pattern of behavior. The greater the sense of individual security, however, the more likely this is to occur.

Actually, the behavior of maladjusted persons does not differ in kind from that of so-called normal persons (which covers a wide range and many sins!). It differs only in degrees. Everyone projects at some time. Some persons project more often than others, and mentally ill patients may project more extensively and even use projection as a major technique in adaptation. The rather shy person who seems quite all right, generally speaking, but refuses an invitation because important persons will be present, is using the same broad pattern of behavior shown by the patient in a state hospital who sits alone in one position, head down, never speaking, and apparently unaware of his surroundings. This similarity between so-called normal behavior and abnormal behavior may be one of the factors that helps to explain to some degree the rejection of the mentally ill persons.

For the sake of convenience, we group behavior into broad patterns which have certain major characteristics in common. However, no two individuals behave *exactly* alike, and no two persons, sick or well, ever duplicate each other. This is eminently reasonable if we but recall the profound possibilities for variations and differences in the organic endowment and the past experiences of people. No situation is exactly the same for any two people since the interaction between environment and organism is most significant, and no two people bring the same selective perception to any given situation. In all this infinite variety it becomes apparent that interpretation of behavior is no easy matter. We cannot easily judge the meaning of an experience for another since we always see it in terms of our own experience. Recognition of this fact is the first step in learning to observe behavior intelligently.

The deviations from the normal range of behavior that indicate sufficient disorganization of the self to render it ineffective in maintaining security in a socially acceptable manner are called mental illnesses. This is the deepest degree of lack of mental health. On a cultural judgment, we tend to separate them into two categories—psychoses and psychoneuroses. The psychoses are generally considered the major mental illnesses, and behavior is thought to be more bizarre and further from contact with reality. The psychoneuroses are considered minor mental illnesses in which the patient retains a closer contact with reality and is better able to get along in society. Actually, the line between the two is indistinct. In addition, a psychoneurosis may well be more permanent than a psychosis. This may possibly be explained by the fact that the significance of the types of behavior shown by so-called neurotic persons is only beginning to be understood and, until recently, have been fairly well accepted by society. The labels minor and major mental illness are not an accurate index of the degree of malignancy of the illness.

The deviations in behavior that occur will be classified roughly for discussion. Insecurity may dominate the feeling tones of many persons, but the particular situation that arouses it and the method of handling the anxiety aroused will be different from person to person. Such method will be an expression of the personality.

Withdrawal

One method of handling the problems of interpersonal relationships is by withdrawal, the purpose of which is protective. By withdrawing and avoiding relationships, an individual avoids further damage to his security. The danger of such a pattern is that it inevitably produces loneliness. Compensations may be developed, but the pattern of avoidance carries over into the compensatory adjustment and thus effectively limits its usefulness. Regression may occur, and the ultimately unsuccessful outcome may be a retreat to infantile levels. In such a stage, thinking becomes once again autistic in nature, that is, highly personal in meaning and not validated or checked by experience or reality.

Withdrawal is manifested in many degrees and may even be quite spotty in its appearance within the personality. Persons may avoid only types of situations in which security has been previously undermined and yet maintain a positive approach to the rest of the experience. For example, a student may do extremely well on every subject except history which he cannot learn. His first history teacher may have been a sarcastic

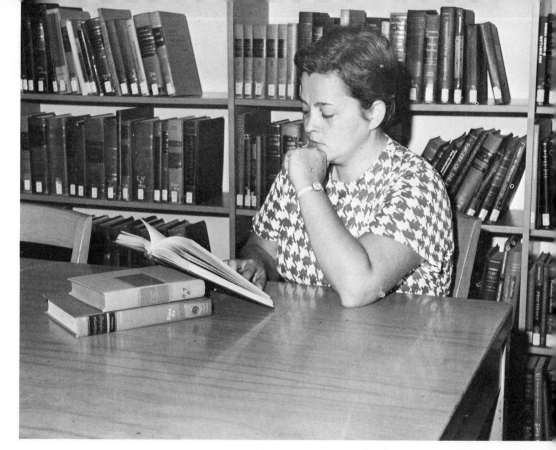

The bookworm can use intellectual interests to isolate self from contact with other people.

person who constantly belittled him, a fact he may not remember at all or may recall with difficulty. This occurrence he does not associate with his inability to master the particular subject. In the process of first studying history, his security was undermined. So, despite what appears to be outward efforts to conform, the unconscious block set up operates to keep him from grasping the fundamentals that would make history easy for him. He avoids coming to grips with it and simply laughingly explains that the subject is too much for him. Most of us have exactly such blind spots.

Withdrawal has many degrees of expression. It may occur only as a temporary or seldom used pattern through various phases to the withdrawn psychotic patient who seems completely indifferent to his environment. (It must be noted that patients never completely lose all contact with reality or all relationships with others, however inadequate those relationships may be.) Withdrawal may be expressed through avoidance of contact with others on every possible occasion or through frequent contact with many different people, with all relationships kept on a superficial level. It may be expressed through quick, violent friendships that come to an early and abrupt end. It may be expressed through the cynical rejection of people as worthless.

When withdrawal begins to dominate the pattern of behavior, loneliness ensues. The organization of the self is headed in the direction of rejection, and self-rejection is reflected in rejection of others. The vicious circle set in motion is hard to break. The potentialities for complete regression are always present, and a crisis in living may precipitate it. The ultimate outcome depends upon the positive attitudes integrated into the self, upon the balance of positive attitudes and powerful motivations in the unconscious and dissociated self, and upon further experience.

Aggression

Aggression is another method of handling the problems of interpersonal relationships, and a frequent pattern for those whose self-perception and hence perception of others is predominantly hostile. The expression of aggression, openly or symbolically, is common to all of us since hostility is a universal experience. When it dominates the personality and the direction of its development, difficulties inevitably ensue. Open aggression may discharge energy, but it calls forth retaliation which carries a threat to security. Again the problem becomes one of a vicious cycle set in motion.

The extent and form of expression of aggression may vary markedly. The sarcastic remark, the unfavorable comments about one relayed "for your own good," the forgetting of names and appointments, and the constant use of ridicule may all be expressions of hostility.

Hostility may be expressed rather frankly and openly toward certain persons, and the individual makes sure that they are aware of the dislike he feels. It may also be expressed as a general contempt for people and for their aspirations, their ambitions, and their opinions. The individual who concentrates always on the weakness of other persons in his perception of them is expressing his hostility toward people in general and himself in particular. This is often seen in the "I love you dearly, BUT—" pattern in which the discussion of the "but" is elaborated with a treatise of one's faults. The "I love you dearly" that prefaces the approach is a screening attempt to prevent retaliation and expresses some fear of reprisal. Hostility is frequently disguised because the person who feels it often does suffer from the fear of retribution.

One of the more subtle forms of hostility results from reaction formation or the development of the exact opposite trait as a compensatory protective device. Here we have the person who is exclusively thoughtful and courteous. Interestingly enough, such people usually make one thoroughly uncomfortable and with good reason, because such is their exact intention. Another outcome, and one that is serious in its implications, is that a strongly hostile perception of existence may arouse so much fear and anxiety within the self lest it find outward expression that it is turned upon the self. Such an inward direction for deep hostility underlies genuine suicidal attempts. Harshly punitive experiences in situations that arouse deep hostility may induce such a pattern. Aggression may also be displaced onto the environment, and an individual may be quite destructive with material objects, consciously or unconsciously. This is usually accompanied, however, by a subtle expression of hostility in interpersonal relations.

The pattern of hostility may relate only to certain types of situations. A staff nurse may get along quite well with students, auxiliary workers, and other staff nurses, but makes life very difficult for those in authority. The pattern of hostility may even be limited to female authority. This is related to previous experiences of circumscribed occurrence which have undermined security and called forth hostility as a response. If sufficient positive attitudes are part of the self, corrective experiences are very likely to be fruitful for personality growth. On the other hand, consistently unfortunate experience in other areas may lead to a spread of the pattern of hostile perceptions.

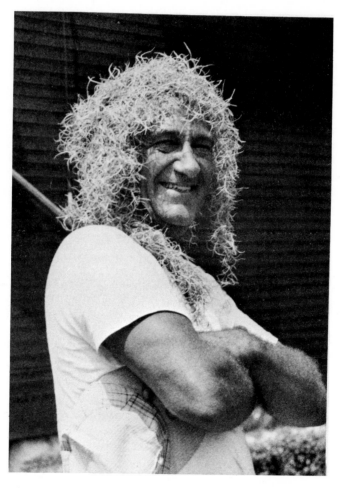

The life of the party has his counterpart in psychopathology in the overactive patient.

The most serious manifestation of this pattern is in the form of mental illness in which impulsive, uncontrolled, aggressive behavior explodes and is usually accompanied by a terrific speeding up of the entire activity of the personality. Verbal and physical aggression are open and frank, interrupted often by a raucous humor that is indication of the enjoyment of such expression. Even in this syndrome, however, the fear of retribution is indicated by flashes of depression or self-punishment, probably in an attempt to avoid punishment from others.

Another serious manifestation is depression, a destructive process whereby the self is severely punished, and its total activity in all areas depressed. These two syndromes may occur in combination or one following the other. It is as though the patient directed his aggression outward and then, having gone so far, develops a fear of serious retribution, and directs his aggression inward to avoid the consequences.

Depressions are thought by many to be due to the experience of loss—be it a loved one, a material object with symbolic significance, or a job. The individual's depressed reaction is due to (1) the behavior pattern established through early experience of loss and (2) the existence of an unconscious wish to punish both the lost object and to punish the self.

Projection

The third pattern of handling the problem of attaining security in interpersonal relationships is projection. As has been pointed out before, this is a common mechanism and one that is used fairly frequently by all of us. The protective function here is obvious. One protects one's sense of security by attributing to others one's own personal faults or one's own personal failures. Listen to the postmortems over a heated disagreement. In ninety cases out of a hundred, the other fellow was wrong. We seldom fail on our own merits, but because someone else usually makes it impossible for us to succeed. The list of traits that arouse a sharply disagreeable reaction in us is usually a list of our own traits of which we are almost always unaware.

Projection is perhaps more easily identifiable than the two previously discussed patterns. It is a little harder to disguise on close acquaintance. It is seen in the practice of excusing failures through blaming the interference of others. It is seen in more serious forms when it develops as a result of certain compensatory conceits to help rebuild the shattered sense of security. These are manifested through an inflated sense of one's own importance and are expressed by referring all environmental happenings as being significant to the self. The pen left carelessly by the secretary on the left side of the desk instead of its usual place on the right has meaning. The secretary is saying, "I'll do as I please; you can't boss me," or "Your character is changing." This process can continue in development until the environmental forces appear to combine into an organized conspiracy against the patient. "The FBI is out to get me." Here we see both the basic self-perception, a negative and hostile self-organization, and the compensatory reaction it produced, an inflated self-conception not founded on reality, but on a self important enough to be of concern to the Federal Bureau of Investigation.

The use of projection rests upon a fundamentally derogatory self-estimate, combined with an active tendency to seek security insistently. The personality carries within itself the seed of its own defeat since it selectively perceives and integrates those parts of experience which are consistent with the self-organization. The derogatory or critical attitude toward the self is expressed in a superior manner and critical attitude toward others, which is often seen in so-called normal behavior through a wide range of behavior with this trait as its central characteristic. The ultimate disorganization is found in the state hospital patient with elaborate ideas about being a very important person who is persecuted and held prisoner in the hospital by the combined forces of the Army, Navy, Marines, Air Force, and John L. Lewis' United Mine Workers.

Use of physical disability

Another devious method of attempting to attain security is by concentration on the physical aspects of existence and the development of certain physical defects or ailments. Here a double purpose is usually accomplished. The individual develops physical infirmities that force him to avoid the types of situations that produce anxiety and reduces the demands likely to be made on him by society. In addition, he secures a certain amount of sympathy because of the physical illness itself. It is also a weapon with which to demand the attention of others. If one doctor finally reaches a limit with the patient when he can find no organic cause for the presenting complaint, there are always other doctors. Fundamentally, such a pattern of behavior is evasive in nature. Its selection as a means of resolving conflicts and protecting the self is usually related closely to early experience. If physical aches and pains were the only method of gaining any sign of affection from parents, that is the pattern likely to be followed in any crisis thereafter. If experience outside the home has confirmed the parents' original evaluation of the child as important only when sick, the pattern becomes fixed. If the stress a developing personality undergoes is severe, the more likely the pattern is to be used. A severe and prolonged physical illness early in life may also serve to focus attention on the workings of the body and may result in a tendency to react to severe stress with the development of some ailment.

Again we find this type of behavior in a wide range of expressions from normal to abnormal. Strong emotions, as any student of physiology knows, have a physical accompaniment. Anxiety is both a physical and emotional phenomenon. A headache before an examination is easy to explain, as is a feeling of nausea at some unpleasant experience. In addition, the majority of us at some time or another, and sometimes more often than others, use physical complaints as a means of evasion. Once in a while it is pure malingering, that is, consciously and with malice aforethought, as when we avoid a dinner we do not want to attend with the excuse of a nonexistent headache. There are, however, many times when we use the alibi unconsciously. We *do* have a headache; yet it miraculously disappears when the hour for the party to begin has passed. Quite virtuously, we go elsewhere and have a good time.

A somewhat more severe instance is the person with a chronic complaint who has it to rely upon when any situation arises which may carry a threat to security. Varying degrees of the use of such behavior exist all the way to the bedridden, paralyzed individual who forces the entire household to organize itself around her needs.

It is an amusing commentary on our culture that one of its major preoccupations in personal life is with the function of the gastrointestinal tract. Nausea and vomiting, diarrhea, and constipation are very common occurrences, important topics for conversation, and accepted alibis for almost anything!

There do occur some substitute processes for physical ailments, such as the circumscribed memory loss that we call amnesia. In function and purpose they are similar to the use of physical ailments to evade and excuse.

As can readily be seen, this pattern of behavior has coherence only through its method of action and the limited aims it sets for satisfactions. Everything is subordinated to the achievement of a precarious security. Its forms of expression can range through the entire manual of medicine. In some cases, prolonged use of physical complaints for psychologic purpose may actually produce somatic illnesses. This usually manages to completely confuse the organic-minded member of the health team.

Use of ritualistic behavior

Another method of handling the problems of interpersonal relationships is through rigidly ritualistic behavior designed to retain control over the situation and keep anxiety at a minimum. This appears most obviously as compulsive acts which *must* be done regardless of how foolish they may seem intellectually to the doer. Stemming from a profound sense of inferiority, the individual responds to a compulsion from outside which is built into a sort of magic operation which gives him security, that is, gives him the sense of control over a situation which is an essential base of security. Usually, compulsive behavior is extremely difficult for others in the environment, and the patient subtly expresses his self-judgment and contempt toward others.

This compulsive-obsessional type of behavior has many expressions. Usually preceding the compulsive act are obsessive ideas, and the normal person shows evidences of both. The song that keeps running through the mind until it becomes annoying is an example. A conscious effort to change the preoccupation usually comes to naught the moment attention is distracted, and one finds oneself humming or singing the recurring song again. After the apartment is locked, some persons *must* go back to make sure the last cigarette was put out or the gas turned off, although the trip back proves unnecessary. The toothbrush *must* be hung up to dry, or sleep is elusive. Ash trays *must* be emptied or anxiety and worry occur. Fundamentally, these are magical operations which dispel a threat by keeping the situation in a certain known sequence which is a form of control over the environment. One is, thereby, in control and therefore secure.

Compulsive-obsessional behavior may occur simply as an occasional episode in normal experience or as a constantly recurring episode in relation to one act or one situation. It may progress to a severe and prolonged ritual which actually severely handicaps a person in his adjustment. One of the best examples is the elaborate ritual of hand washing of the very compulsive patient. Every time his hands touch something, he must wash them. It is believed this represents a cleansing in a symbolic sense, that it controls anxiety aroused by a sense of guilt that exists in the dissociated self or unconscious. It is controlled by a symbolic act, or by magic. The individual who must wash his hands every time they touch something has not enough time left to hold a job.

Props that blur reality

Another method of handling personal problems is to blur reality with some outside influence that either changes the nature of reality or enhances one's sense of the ability to deal with it. Morphine, for example, produces in the individual a delightful sense of well-being that can only be matched by the attainment of complete biologic satisfaction with a maximum of social approval. For those whose attainment of security is difficult because of difficulties in personality development, this artificial attainment may well become a prop on which they can lean. Alcohol and various other drugs may offer the same false security. Recovery from their effects enhances the lack of security and leads to a renewal of and dependence on their use. This resolution of conflicts seems to be typical of persons whose tolerance for anxiety and frustration is very low.

Failure to integrate

The final method is probably the least understood of all. We can do no more than describe it. This consists of *failing* to integrate experience so that the past counts only as it indicates positively the future to an observer; yet the past and future have little significance for the individual himself. He neither profits from past experience nor takes account of future consequences. Verbally, he is fluent and often superficially charming, but depth and duration of emotion are alien to him. He lives purely for the moment, reaching out to satisfy predominantly biologic satisfactions with little concern for enduring personal security. What produces him we do not know; how to alter his behavior or expose him to corrective experience is a puzzle.

Deviations of organic origin

The techniques of behavior we have previously discussed are at the present time considered functional in origin although recent discoveries in biochemistry raise some questions about this. There are no organic or somatic changes that will account for their appearance. Other types of maladjustment severe enough to be considered mental illness do originate in damage to the central nervous system, which is the system most influential in the coordination of the behavior of a human being into a unitary response. When such damage does occur, there are usually specific symptoms which indicate the area involved, plus an accentuation, uncontrolled in type, of the basic personality of the individual. For example, the gray cells are destroyed in syphilitic invasion of the cerebral cortex. The powers of association and fine muscular coordination, the ability to calculate, and the ability to remember accurately, dependent upon cortex cells, are destroyed. In addition to these symptoms a breakdown in personality may occur, and its direction will be determined by the direction of the personality previous to the organic damage. A hostile person will show a disorder characterized by hostility; a withdrawn person will show a disorder characterized by withdrawal; and so forth. The end result is always a fusion of organic, intellectual, and emotional components.

Summary

This chapter has shown some of the ways in which behavior can deviate from the accepted social pattern and has given brief indications of the sources of such deviations. Early experience, as has been indicated, is extremely important for the direction and growth of personality and the attainment of mental health. If experience builds a healthy respect for the self that permits the more powerful motivational systems direct access to consciousness and therefore satisfaction without serious threat to security, the chances of mental illness are low. The more powerful the motivational systems that are forced by painful or traumatic experience into the dissociated or unconscious part of the self, the greater will be the danger of acute disruptions of the personality. The degree of mental health is related closely to awareness of one's motivations as balanced by the depth of stresses to which the individual is exposed. By this is meant not merely intellectual insight but emotional acceptance of that insight also. The motivations recognized must be acceptable to the perception of one's self. A person must be able to live comfortably with his weaknesses, and his strengths must be reasonably well assessed.

References

Brown, Myrtle Irene: Socialization: A social theory of adaptation, Nursing Science 1:280-294, Oct.-Nov. 1963.

Cameron, Norman: The psychology of behavior disorders, New York, 1947, Houghton Mifflin Co., pp. 103-186.

Frazier, Shervert and Carr, Arthur C.: Introduction to psychopathology, New York, 1964, The Macmillan Co.

Peplau, Hildegarde E.: Interpersonal relationships and the process of adaptation, Nursing Science 1:272-279, Oct.-Nov. 1963.

Sullivan, Harry Stack: Conceptions of modern psychiatry, Washington, D. C., 1947, William Alanson White Psychiatric Foundation, pp. 43-86.

Chapter vi

Basic approaches
to psychiatric therapy

A s pointed out before, a unified concept of mental health and mental disease has not yet been developed. The specific causes of and specific cures for specific mental illnesses are not known. It is not surprising, therefore, to find the simultaneous existence of a variety of approaches to the provision of therapy for patients. Sometimes the variations seems to rest more on differences in emphasis than on real disagreement about the nature of man and the factors that determine how he learns to change his behavior. Certain common threads of agreement exist among the varied schools of thought. Among practically all therapeutic approaches the use of diagnosis has shifted from emphasizing classification into categories of illness to focusing upon the particular problems of the patient.

Since schools of therapy have mutliplied, above and beyond the variations in the psychoanalytic schools, no attempt will be made to present all of them in this brief discussion. A random sample of current varying approaches will be reviewed purely to indicate and make understandable the fact of variation and some of its implications for patient care, including nursing care. Some of the schools presented are basically psychoanalytic in origin and orientation.

Variations in theoretical approaches

In a preceding chapter, some of the basic concepts in psychoanalysis and their variations in different schools of thought were presented. The method of treatment used is also called psychoanalysis and has as its goal the complete personality reconstruction of the patient through self-understanding of past problems, attitudes, and behaviors and their influence on present behavior. While there are variations in the field of practice, the standard or classic technique is built upon the patient's active participation through free association, the expression of whatever thoughts occur. Resistances to free association develop and are interpreted to the patient. The patient brings to and acts out again in his relationship with his therapist the attitudes and behavior patterns experienced in past relationships, and these are interpreted to him. Thus the misinterpretation of the present in terms of the past is resolved by interpretation. Basic to the therapeutic process is the "transference neurosis" in which the patient transfers to the therapist past attitudes and relationships. The ultimate goal of therapy is the full development, understanding, and resolution of the transference neurosis. Basic therapeutic factors are emotional abreaction, intellectual insight, and the recovery of repressed infantile memories.

In contrast to the psychoanalytic emphasis upon past experiences, the psychobiologic school, founded by Adolf Meyer, places an emphasis upon analysis by the patient of present situations and their meaning and present attitudes. Meyer called his approach "distributive analysis and synthesis." Under the guidance of the therapist, the patient attempts to identify the dynamic factors underlying his behavior. This is largely done at the conscious level, using inductive reasoning and discussion to develop an understanding which can be used to change patterns of behavior in a constructive direction. The patient's current problems and unhealthy emotional attitudes form the basis of analysis rather than the patient-physician relationship.

The "adaptational theory" of personality development was primarily the work of Rado, Kardiner, and Levy. They see the integrating factor that unifies the self as arising from behavior goals or motivations aroused by internal physiologic needs or external cultural demands. When needs arise, real or fantasied, action results, with the self-image increased or decreased in terms of success of the action. The self-image is rooted in the individual's interpretation of his ability to satisfy his needs. Adaptation is viewed as the relationship of means to ends, that is, the efficiency of the individual in meeting his goals. This school interprets development as going through three stages, related to the level of central nervous system organization. The first level is the pain-pleasure level, with motivation related to the need for release from physical or psychologic tension. Anticipation and foresight have not yet been developed. The emotional level is the succeeding stage, and emotion rather than instinct is considered the major integrating force in behavior. Love, grief, fear, and rage are the primary emotional forces. Foresight and anticipation are added at this level. Self-centeredness is also characteristic of this level. The final stage of development is the rational aspect of man—thought. On this level, as emotion is to some extent replaced by thought, man becomes capable of objectivity, and his perception of reality changes. It should be remembered that reason does not fully dominate man's reactions, and emotion and thought interchangeably hold the upper hand. For example, emotional thought is considered basic to the occurrence of psychopathology and is aroused by the perception of danger, real or fantasied. When anxiety is aroused, riddance (rejection or denial) and repression operate to control the anxiety, restricting the self. The resulting inhibition and avoidance are basic to the use of neurotic behavior patterns.

This school also holds that the early formative years are extremely important for later life. In the development of his self-image, the infant begins as an omnipotent, egocentric being endowed with magical power. As reality impinges, the sense of omnipotence is transferred to the parents, and the need arises to mold behavior to remain in their good graces. This leads to a further deepening of the impact of reality, and the appearance of critical thinking brings about self-observation and self-criticism. An ideal self or ego-ideal develops, usually through the process of identification, and the ideal self is an integrative factor in the socialization of the individual. This ego-ideal is derived from the attitudes and feelings of significant persons in the immediate environment. The self then moves onward to the internalization of the values of the society in which he lives. Repressed aspects of life influence the functions of the self from the unconscious, and such emotionally charged needs, denied access to awareness, may distort reality perception. The adaptational school emphasizes the indestructibility of infantile omnipotence and its potential for revival. Therapy in this school has two approaches—reparative and reconstructive. Reparative therapy is short-term, designed to provide support for the patient to help him deal with the immediate situation, helping him to function more comfortably. Reparative therapy utilizes support, emotional release, persuasion or suggestion, direct intervention, and superficial insight. Reconstructive therapy aims beyond this to both an intellectual understanding of the meaning of ones' own behavior and an insight, or acceptance, that leads to behavior changes. The patient-physician relationship is considered the basic method in both types of therapy.

Roy Grinker, one of the major supporters of the transactional school, has proposed an approach to psychiatric therapy based upon an operational theory of psychotherapy rather than upon psychodynamics or diagnosis. It is based upon field theory, role theory, and communication theory. From the field theory is taken the significance of the environmental setting and its meaning, explicit and implicit, for both the patient and the therapist. This includes, above and beyond the particular institutional situation, the social environments, both past and present, of both participants. Both aspects of the environment will have their influence on the therapeutic process. Explicit roles are those the individual learned from society about his accepted patterns of behavior with certain categories of other people. All individuals have varying roles they carry out with varying people. For example, a person interchangeably behaves as a mother, a daughter, a friend, or a teacher. Such roles are usually easily identified. Expectations of the behavior of others is also influenced by the concept of the other's role. Implicit roles, on the other hand, are aspects of the individual's own complexity, usually remote from awareness and consciousness, reflect early identifications, and are not easily made explicit. Roles with other people are most comfortable when they complement each other. Grinker proposes that roles, explicit and implicit, in the two-person group of patient-therapist be regarded as interacting roles, and therapy then involves behavior of a person in terms of his role in reaction with the therapist. Such roles are expressed by communication, verbal and nonverbal. Communication is subject to distortion—as communication clears and distortion disappears, therapy progresses. Thus, two individuals in a specific environment, each affecting the other and reacting to each other's response feedbacks, transact in a reciprocal, cyclical, and everchanging process.

The transactionalist, in therapy, does not focus upon early experiences, memories, or relationships, but deals with the here-and-now communication between the patient and therapist about their relationship. The development of a transference neurosis is avoided if possible. The goal of therapy is broadly to help the patient back to health, and the specific goals develop as therapy progresses. The transactional school also uses the interview technique, but places a somewhat different emphasis upon the therapist's role. The desire to help and to understand is considered an essential basic attitude of the therapist, and this does agree with other schools of thought. Permissiveness encourages patient verbal expression, but does not carry over to acting out. The therapist, however, takes an active role, choosing focus, avoiding silences, and controlling the interview. He declines to assume the implicit roles in which the patient tries to place him. He is also honest about expressing his own feelings and, if he is angry, says so. The impassive, imperturbable role is not for the therapist of the transactional school.

The existential school of psychology and psychiatry (Rollo May is one of its better known exponents) places its approach to therapy upon existential philosophy. This emphasizes the understanding of a phenomenon as it exists, rather than trying to explain the nature of people or existence by their causes. It is less "why" a thing is than "what" a thing is that is significant. Such a belief leads logically to more emphasis upon what the patient is as a person than how he got that way. This approach also stresses that all ways of understanding man are based upon assumptions which need examination. Some of the basic beliefs about man that underlie the existential theories of psychotherapy include the following.

1. All people are potentially centered in themselves.
2. People need and strive to preserve their center.
3. People have the possibility and need to go out from their centeredness and participate in relations with others.
4. The human being possesses a distinctively human form of awareness—self consciousness, the awareness that I am I.
5. The unconscious consists of experience that the person cannot let himself fully experience in awareness.
6. Anxiety and guilt, potentially tragic, are necessary concomitants of the conscious awareness of the self as a responsible being.
7. Anxiety and guilt are not wholly negative.
8. The capacity to confront death (the tragic aspect of life) is prerequisite to growth, self-discovery, and full self-consciousness.

In this view, neurotic reactions are seen as modes of adjustment, however restricted, rather than maladaptations. The central goal of personality becomes conscious, realistic knowledge of one's self and the courage to face one's own destiny as a responsible person. Therapy is concerned less with removing or reducing anxiety and guilt than with learning how to live with normal anxiety and guilt. Neurotic anxiety and guilt are characterized by inappropriateness, repression into the unconscious, symptom formation, and destructiveness. The basic goal of psychotherapy is to provide the patient with a relationship (or encounter) in which he can confront his anxiety and guilt and turn them from neurotic to normal and learn to accept and tolerate his real self.

The client-centered therapeutic school, associated with the name of its founder Carl Rogers, has had a considerable impact upon psychiatric nursing. Certain basic tenets, that underlie the approach of Rogers and his associates to therapy are the following.

1. Basic personality orientation is always in the direction of health.
2. The focus of therapy is on the present.
3. Personality development and the process of therapy exist upon a continuum from unawareness of feelings and experiencing to awareness of and trust in feeling and experience.
4. A healthy self-concept rests upon integrating and accepting all aspects of the self.
5. Personality change toward health can result from a helping relationship.
6. The essence of a helping relationship consists of providing (1) unconditional and nonpossessive liking, (2) an attitude of trying to understand feelings and experience as they seem to the patient, and (3) congruence, that is, consistency between the helper's verbalizations and behavior and real feelings.

Rogers identifies seven stages in personality development and the process of therapy and has elaborated these in regard to feelings and personal meanings, manner of experiencing, congruence, and communication of self. In the area of feelings and personal meanings, the seven developmental stages are as follows.

1. Unawareness
2. Described as external to self
3. Described as past
4. Described as present, owned by self
5. Freely expressed
6. Those previously denied awarenesses, experienced immediately and accepted
7. Owned and accepted and trusted as behavior guides

The seven stages in the manner of experiencing are as follows.

1. Meaning of experience in the past
2. Reacts as though experience in the past
3. Described as in the past

4. Unwilling recognition of experiencing
5. Conceptualization and expression
6. Acceptance of process of experiencing
7. Comfortable with changing flow of experience

The seven stages in the area of congruence are as follows.

1. Unaware of discrepancies between experience and awareness
2. Contradictory statements about self
3. Contradictions recognized
4. Concern expressed about contradictions
5. Contradictions recognized as different aspects of personality
6. Experiences change from incongruence to congruence
7. Acceptance of varying aspects of self

A similar seven-stage development covers moving from the inability to communicate the self to full awareness and communication of internal experiencing.

Based upon studies and experience, Rogers has suggested it may be possible to analyze and study people and patients in relation to his theory of the continuum in personality development and the process of therapy rather than through patient history, personality type, or diagnosis.

A more recent approach to therapy, directed toward the family as a unit rather than toward the patient as an individual, is in the process of testing a theoretic basis for family therapy. Nathan W. Ackerman is one of its best known exponents. The intimate relationship of the personality development of the infant and child to family equilibrium or disequilibrium is so firmly entrenched that therapy for disturbed children automatically includes work with parents or their surrogates. Ackerman believes the family significance for adolescent and adult personality function is equally important, and he suggests we need a broader basis than we currently have for the theory of personality development and adult functioning. The family group (those who live under one roof) can make or break mental health since the family constitutes the unit of living and the unit of experience. The family group shapes personal adaptation within the family and outside the family, not merely in childhood but throughout life. The family as a unit has an identity of its own, not always easy to pinpoint because it is dynamic and undergoes continuous change. But the family identity and its relationship to mental illness and mental health are worth study.

The extent to which a family supports mental health is apparent on three levels—the psychiatric illness of one or more of its members, the control of anxiety and thereby the prevention of outright breakdown, and the positive promotion of growth and creativity. The family interrelationships are primary factors in determining the extent to which its members can maintain stability, tolerate new experience, and learn to change and grow. The balance between stability and the capacity to learn and grow represents the essence of homeostasis of behavior. The balance of role relationships within the family may or may not (1) satisfy personal needs, (2) provide means of solving conflicts, (3) support tolerable self-images, and (4) provide support for anxiety defenses in related members. The degree to which the family as a unit does this positively or negatively is an index of its contribution, positive or negative, to mental health.

The therapeutic technique utilized by the family therapist is the interview, but the interview is with the total family, that is, all who live under one roof. The role of the therapist includes promoting awareness and honest expression of feelings, activating hope, challenging or identifying defense operations, and maintaining control so that anxiety and aggression do not explode. The therapist is directive, forthright, and frank, and permits himself to be drawn into the center of the family disturbance; he remains impartial but never neutral. In addition, the therapist interacts with all, and while he may have favorites, these shift from member to member of the family. The family-interview approach uses transference, resistance, and interpretation, but in a modified setting.

By now, group psychotherapy has become an established and accepted therapeutic method. Its rapid development since World War II is probably related to the shortage of psychiatrists and the increased recognition of the need for therapeutic help on the part of many persons, mentally ill or otherwise. Its theoretic orientation is varied, since the theoretic background of the therapist may be in almost any of the varying schools of psychiatric and/or psychologic thought. Once used purely as an adjunct to individual psychotherapy, group psychotherapy is now the treatment of choice for many patients. Underlying this approach is the concept that anxiety and guilt are aroused in relation to other people and in a social setting, and it is in such a setting that a changed personality organization can best be achieved. The group is also considered a family substitute, and some of its value is thought to derive from this. Group psychotherapy also emphasizes the contribution the patient himself makes to the therapy of others and himself through mutual interpretation and support. In general, groups focus on the encouragement of free and honest expression of feelings, interpretation of individual reactions and group interaction, and the honest dealing with problems. The activity of the therapist is guided by his theoretic orientation.

Running through all the therapeutic approaches are certain commonalities. All schools emphasize the helping relationship, individual or group, and the need for the therapist to convey a genuine desire to help and to understand his patient or patients. All schools emphasize the influence of the therapist as a person upon his patient and upon the process of therapy. In addition, all approaches recognize the centrality of anxiety and its avoidance as vital motivators in behavior. All concede the overwhelming importance of the unconscious. The importance for mental health of the individual's self-image or self-concept is also universal. All schools show more concern with mental illness than with mental health. All schools lean heavily upon the interview technique, and all schools rest to some extent on the foundations of psychoanalytic concepts.

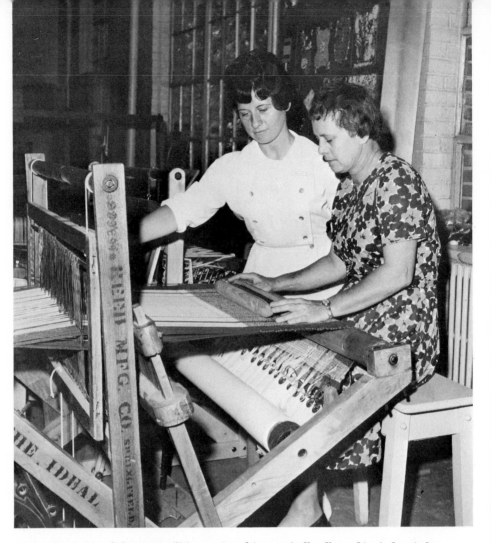

Occupational therapy facilities are found in practically all psychiatric hospitals.

Nonspecific therapeutic approaches

The therapeutic approaches discussed in the previous section represent theoretic bases upon which intensive individual or group psychotherapy are practiced. The majority of hospitalized psychiatric patients do not receive such psychotherapy, but exist in settings where certain practices are considered generally therapeutic, regardless of the patient's particular problem, age, sex, or any other factor that would be taken into consideration in individual therapy. Such broad therapeutic assumptions influence hospital setting, organization, and functions.

One of the basic therapeutic assumptions is that activity at least prevents regression and at best helps promote recovery. In the latter, activity provides both reality contact and an opportunity to practice or to develop social skills. This is a long cherished concept, and it accounts for the numerous activity programs found in most psychiatric hospitals. It has led to the utilization of a number of departments or programs—occupational therapy, recreational therapy, social therapy (such as dances and movies), work details, art therapy, and workshops, for example. The pervasive influence of the idea that activity is of therapeutic value is easy to recognize in most institutional psychiatric settings.

Somewhat harder to recognize in most large institutional mental hospitals, but easily recognizable in new psychiatric hospitals is the therapeutic assumption that the physical environment has an impact upon and can contribute to patient therapy. Surroundings that are cheerful and that approximate social settings outside the hospital are at present considered desirable. Many efforts at improving the physical appearance of patient care units have been accompanied by improved patient behavior. Whether this results from improved patient morale or improved staff morale remains a moot point. In either case, it is a generally accepted belief that the physical environment is a therapeutic instrument.

Another generally accepted assumption, although not always acted upon, is that nonrestraint is therapeutic. History would appear to support this thesis. When Pinel struck the chains from patients, patient behavior improved. The spreading open-door policy in psychiatric hospitals is a resurgance of an old idea. New variations in treatment go somewhat beyond nonrestraint and include giving the patient more responsibility, as in patient government.

Another broad assumption is that aspects of the basic helping relationship can be constructively assumed by all personnel who come in contact with patients. This concept, too, is not a new one, but is being revived with greater emphasis. Physicians spend more time working with and through other team members, and physicians and nurses spend more time working with attendants or aides, helping them toward greater understanding of the patients for whom they provide care. Nursing education generally is trying to prepare its practitioners at all levels for more effective use of the helping relationship.

Another basic therapeutic assumption, and one that is only beginning to receive real attention, is that the working relationship among the personnel who care for patients is also a therapeutic tool. It has been conclusively demonstrated that covert conflict among personnel leads to regressed behavior on the part of patients. That cooperative working relationships lead to a similar impact, but positive in nature, has not been as clearly demonstrated.

That the social structure, and especially the implicit social goals, of the setting in which a patient finds himself is a therapeutic tool is another basic assumption. If the personnel group goal is centered on patient control, the patient suffers. If the personnel group goal is focused on patient recovery or improvement, patient behavior improves.

Another basic therapeutic assumption is that patient interaction with other people, staff or other patients or visitors, contributes to recovery possibilities. This assumption underlies the many efforts in and outside the patient care unit to provide the opportunity for and to encourage patient interaction with others. One of the major responsibilities of the nurse in the psychiatric hospital is to promote patient socialization.

Through all of the nonspecific therapeutic approaches, current trends are emphasizing active patient participation and increased patient responsibility for himself. Another current trend of significance is an increased understanding of the impact of expectations of patient behavior on such behavior and, consequently, conscious efforts to improve personnel expectations of patient behavior.

Somatic approaches to therapy

Throughout the history of psychiatric therapy, the somatic treatment of mental illness has been an approach that has been explored from many points of view. For example, before the advent of penicillin, syphilis of the central nervous system was treated by fever therapy, often the use of malaria. We have just recently completed the shock era, in which electroconvulsive therapy and insulin shock were widely used. The major somatic approach today is found in chemotherapy or the use of the tranquilizers. Their advent has had a profound impact on mental hospitals, since control problems have been sharply reduced and patients are more accessible for the use of interpersonal relationship skills.

In addition to chemotherapy, shock treatment continues to be used, but to a lesser extent. Psychosurgery (severing of association tracts in the brain) is still used to a limited extent. Hydrotherapy is still in use in many psychiatric hospitals.

Specific somatic procedures with their nursing care will be discussed in a later chapter.

References

Frazier, Shervert H. and Karr, Arthur C.: Introduction to psychopathology, New York, 1964, Macmillan Co.

Linn, Louis: Hospital psychiatry. In Arieti, Silvano The American handbook of psychiatry, ed. 2, New York, 1959, Basic Books, Inc., pp. 1829-1839.

Mullan, Hugh and Rosenbaum, Max: Group psychotherapy, New York, 1962, The Free Press of Glencoe.

Noyes, Arthur P. and Kolb, Lawrence C.: Modern clinical psychiatry, ed. 6, Philadelphia, 1963, W. B. Saunders Co., pp. 500-523.

Stein, Morris I., editor: Contemporary psychotherapies, New York, 1961, The Free Press of Glencoe.

Principles of
psychiatric nursing

Chapter vii

Nursing care through understanding

How any one person will behave toward another will depend upon his interpretation of the second person's behavior. One frame of reference used in such interpretation is the cultural setting in which the behavior occurs and the resulting stereotypes it invokes. Another frame of reference is the experiential background of the interpreter which influences his concept of himself in relation to the other person. For example, suppose a young American nurse meets her first mentally ill patient, a patient who is complaining bitterly about the persecutions he is undergoing. She will, in all probability, experience some fear, some uncertainty, some discomfort, and some curiosity or fascination and retreat from the situation. These are typically American attitudes toward mental illness, attitudes which are fortunately undergoing change. If she were a nurse in a culture in which mental illness was considered evidence of divinity, her reaction would probably be one of awe and reverence. On the other hand, suppose she were an experienced and competent psychiatric nurse. She would probably identify the patient's symptom, understand its source, and move to meet the need expressed. In each of these instances, the nurse's response would differ because of the differences in interpretation of the patient's behavior. In other words, what the nurse believes to be the reason for the patient's behavior is an important factor in the response made to it. The nurse's own behavior is one of the most important therapeutic tools she possesses, and its effectiveness is increased as she brings greater understanding to bear on why people behave as they do.

In the care of patients with emotional problems, it is extremely important for the nurse to keep seeking the why behind the patients' behavior without projecting her own reaction to the patient. The why that is important is the why as seen from the patient's point of view, rather than from the nurse's. It is a why that must necessarily be sought objectively.

69

The ability to meet the emotional needs of a patient with a personality disorder is largely dependent upon the ability to understand why he behaves as he does without clouding the conclusion with one's own feelings. Through an analysis of the patient's behavior as an expression of his needs the goals in nursing care are defined. The eternal why, why, why must be applied again and again and again until the general pattern of a patient's behavior spells out the kind of corrective experience he needs to help him toward mental health.

Interpersonal relationships with patients are a definite therapeutic tool and have a real effect on the course of a patient's illness. They can be as efficacious as morphine in the treatment of pain—or they can be sand and salt rubbed on open wounds. Our own behavior toward patients must be directed by an intelligent understanding of why they behave as they do and of what purpose or purposes their behavior may accomplish. We must therefore develop skill in objectively identifying the why of patient behavior.

One of the easiest errors into which we fall, and a very common one, is the acceptance of superficial reasons for behavior that tell us really very little about another person. A patient refuses to cooperate "because he is mean." Granted—but *why* is he mean? Does he need to hurt others, and if so, why? Does he see all other persons as a threat to himself and need to strike first, and if so, why? Is he bitter and cynical, expecting little from others and willing to give less, and if so, why? How deeply and how objectively we reach for that all-important why will govern, to some extent, how we will define the patient's needs and how we will treat him as a person. If we accept him as mean and go no farther, we may fall into the error of trying to teach him for his own good that meanness does not pay dividends. If we see him as one who has been deeply hurt, we can realize the necessity for avoiding further hurt and offering him a relationship that is safe and secure and at the same time realize that by the very depth of his hurt he will need such a relationship for a long time in order to trust it. Either approach will have a very definite effect upon the patient, but one will be detrimental and one may be helpful.

A patient spends his entire time sitting quietly with his head bowed, showing little interest in anything or anyone. He does as he is told, slowly and without interest. At times he appears a little annoyed when anyone talks to him or wants him to do anything. He is completely indifferent to personal appearance although he will passively allow someone to dress him and comb his hair. Why? What purpose can such behavior serve— what does it accomplish? And why is that particular purpose important to the patient?

The most obvious effect of the patient's behavior is to reduce to the lowest possible level any relationships with other persons. He seeks no one. He either passively accepts others in a fashion that gets rid of them as quickly as possible or shows annoyance designed to drive them away. He may be living comfortably in a phantasy world of his own, or he may be quietly and miserably living alone, preferring his lonely misery to the greater one of association with others. What his behavior accomplishes (his purpose) is isolation from other persons.

Man is a social animal, and his social needs are deep-seated and powerful motivating factors in behavior. Security in social relationships is a need that influences all that we are and all that we do. Yet, here is a person who, while seeming quite passive and indifferent, uses those very traits actively to keep himself away from other people and to keep them away from him. We know then that the patient's insecurity in interpersonal relations is so severe that it has overwhelmed him. He feels safer turning his back on real life and real people. In other words, he is defending himself by blocking off any experience which could possibly threaten his self-esteem or which could hurt him in any way. Obviously, the challenge of emotional relationships of any kind with others is something feared. This is a phenomenon very commonly seen in normal life. Many sensitive persons refuse to compete for fearing of losing because the prospective loss will hurt sufficiently to make the gamble and the chance of winning not worth the effort. The self-effacing person who is afraid to voice an opinion is no stranger to any of us. The patient, however, has carried the reaction to extremes. In general, then, he is an individual so deeply insecure in interpersonal relationships that he defends himself by completely rejecting them.

What does the patient's pattern of behavior tell us of his perception of himself in relation to others? We know that his self-confidence is practically nonexistent and can therefore surmise that he feels extremely inferior in comparison to others or may see others in some sense as a very definite threat to himself and his self-esteem. This may well be as far as we can go in general terms from what the patient has shown us in his behavior. Much more specific estimates in terms of how the patient perceives himself can be made when the patient's social history is known and more time has been spent with him. The basic information to begin planning his nursing care, however, is at hand through understanding what the patient's behavior tells us about him. The previously described behavior tells us these significant facts: the patient needs relationships that reassure him as to his worth, that carry absolutely no threat, judgment, or criticism of him, and that will be present long enough and consistently enough to give him an opportunity to accept others. We know he will make it difficult for anyone who tries to help him by rejecting them, by looking for incidents that confirm his fear, and by not knowing how to respond if he wishes to do so. Allowances for the patient's inability to accept help quickly must be made in planning to bolster his weakened ego.

A second patient is extremely restless, physically overactive, and irritable. She is easily distracted by persons or events in her environment and expends a great deal of energy flitting from activity to activity. She "takes over" for other patients and is quite interfering. Waiting on other patients, instructing them in what to do and when to do it, and fighting their battles against personnel are frequent occurrences. In fact, her rare assaultive episodes occur when she intervenes for other patients. She has little liking for personnel and is very sarcastic and supercilious toward them. Placing nurses, doctors, or other staff members in an embarrassing position gives the patient great pleasure, and she exploits such occasions to the fullest without mercy. Along with the constant activity, the patient frequently shows periods of mounting tension which culminate with a loud verbal outburst, almost invariably directed toward personnel. At such times, the patient is markedly crude and profane. What does this behavior accomplish?

The constant activity serves as an outlet for tension to some extent, but its restlessly changing focus and shifting interest make it seem almost as though the patient were afraid to stay with or come to grips with any problem or real purpose. In other words, it is a screen, a block that keeps other things submerged. In much the same way, hard physical activity can be used by the so-called normal person to keep from thinking about unpleasant matters. One thing the patient's behavior certainly accomplishes is to keep him so active and distracted that it diverts him from the normal course of events. It defends him from some situation or emotion that he fears. That the fear is not wholly relieved is indicated by the patient's obvious continued tension. The threat, whatever it may be, is still close.

Another obvious purpose of the patient's behavior is to make personnel as uncomfortable as possible. Hostility is rather frankly expressed. On exactly what grounds the patient's hostility is aroused may not be entirely clear, but there are several possible reasons for it. In a hospital situation, personnel represent authority, and the patient's feeling may stem from hostility toward authority. Or perhaps the fact that personnel are "sane" may make the patient feel uncomfortable enough to arouse her resentment. Her sarcasm, ridicule, and superciliousness may be directed toward reducing personnel to or below the patient's own status. Whatever the basic reason, the patient's behavior expresses her need to strike at the persons who control her environment. Personnel are a sharp threat to her, strong enough to call for attack.

The patient's attitude and behavior toward other patients is also of significance. Although she does not attack them nor express hostility toward them, she does not accept them as being on the same level as herself. She "takes care" of them, she "directs" them, and she "defends" them. She relates herself to other patients by showing an interest in them in a condescending manner. She assumes a superior-inferior status with herself always in the superior role.

The patient's behavior then has two purposes which can be deciphered simply on the basis of observation. She is first of all actively engaged in keeping at bay something that threatens her. In addition, her behavior contributes to her own self-esteem through attacks on personnel that reduce them in stature and through placing herself in a superior relationship to others in the environment. The patient is frantically and consistently trying to increase her sense of importance in her own eyes.

The patient's behavior tells us then that her perception of herself in relation to other persons is that of an individual threatened by everyone with whom she comes in contact. Her greatest threat, calling forth open hostility, is from persons in authority or persons who are higher in the social hierarchy than herself. The patient needs to develop sufficient self-confidence to enable her to be comfortable with other people.

Retaliation against the patient's expressed hostility will confirm her fear of danger and strengthen her need for the elaborate defense she has built. The problem becomes to build the patient's self-confidence slowly and steadily and to avoid any threat, psychologic or physical, directed toward her. Fundamentally, the ultimate objective in caring for this patient is the same as for the first. The difference in the nursing care of the two patients is the difference in the type of obstacles the patient's behavior places on the road to achievement of the nursing goal.

A third patient is completely preoccupied with nonexistent heart trouble. She is forever taking her pulse, suffering from palpitation, heart pain, poor circulation, inability to breathe, etc. She objects strenuously to any activity because of her illness, and she is interested only in her illness. She talks of nothing else. A thorough physical work-up has ruled out definitely any organic pathologic condition. This latter fact only convinces her of the incompetence of the medical staff, and she wishes to be transferred to another hospital. What does this behavior accomplish?

First, why do people tend to sympathize with physical illness? Because it is physically uncomfortable and because physical illness cuts us off from the usual pleasures and pains of everyday existence. These are the important reasons for sympathy. The chronic invalid is limited in his participation in social experience, and this is his greatest tragedy.

The physical complaints without adequate somatic cause accomplish one thing definitely—they limit the range of the patient's experience. If one is ill, there are not only reasons why one cannot do many things ordinarily expected of the average person, but also reasons that are socially acceptable. A person with poor health cannot be expected to work hard for a living. The patient's behavior then is defensive in purpose. It provides him with a means of evading many situations, and when one evades, it is usually because of fear of failure. The patient's concentration upon his heart disease permits him to think well of himself despite the fact that he is not accomplishing anything very constructive or useful to win the approval of his fellow men. He cannot be expected to do much since he is ill.

A person who evades is a person afraid of the consequences. Preoccupied with his own health, the patient is unable to establish and maintain adequate interpersonal relationships with others. He lacks confidence in himself in relation to others to such a degree that he avoids the thing he fears. He compromises with life and settles for a temporary sympathy. He perceives himself as an individual incapable of success and inferior to others and defends himself from the same opinion from others by evasion and alibi. The root of his difficulties is his lack of confidence in himself, and his restoration to health will be synonymous with a growth in his own opinion of himself.

A patient is admitted to a general hospital for major abdominal surgery. She complains that the hospital bed is hard and the sheets are not clean enough. She wants to see her doctor immediately and is annoyed when he is not promptly produced. She criticizes her preparation. She wants water—she wants a bed pan—she wants to go to the bathroom—she wants the head of the bed raised—she wants the head of the bed lowered—she wants the blind raised—she wants the window open—she wants the window closed—and so on, ad infinitum. What on earth can such behavior accomplish except to drive personnel to the contemplation of justifiable homicide?

Two accomplishments stand out when such behavior is viewed objectively. First and most important, the behavior brings other persons to the patient's side. The patient is reaching with poor technique but fervent need for reassurance. Unable to acknowledge it out loud, the patient is frightened and very much needs understanding, tolerance, and reassurance that do not brush aside her fears as unimportant or unnecessary.

Second, criticism of everything in the hospital indicates the patient's uneasiness and makes her feel a little more comfortable by attacking her environment. The criticism underlines the patient's fear and her idea that the hospital is not a place where she is safe and secure. She is not a nasty dispositioned nuisance—she is a very frightened woman. Her perception of herself is the perception of a person in deadly danger.

The development of the ability to understand the implications of patient behavior is essential if the nurse's response is to contribute to the patient's recovery. Nursing care through understanding is the heart of psychiatric nursing—it is the very core of the art of nursing itself for that matter. It is a skill developed only through discipline and constant practice. With every patient the pertinent questions should be asked and reasonable answers sought. What does the patient's behavior accomplish? Why is this purpose important to the patient? How does the patient judge himself as a person? Having reached a tentative conclusion on these important points, the nurse should then try as tactfully as possible to help the patient help himself toward the accomplishment of his purposes in a healthier manner. To do so tactfully means that the nurse must learn to guess intelligently at *what experience means to the patient, not to herself.* A promotion can be a source of satisfaction to one person, a stimulating challenge to another, a threat to a third, and a precipitating factor in a mental illness to a fourth. Intelligent nursing requires not merely that a nurse can imagine herself in another person's situation and visualize how she would feel there, but also that a nurse can imagine herself in another person's situation and visualize how *he* feels.

Constant practice and the readiness and willingness to revise conclusions can help in developing the art of understanding the meaning of experience to others. Judgments should not be based on isolated instances but on the patient's general pattern of behavior as revealed in many situations. Superficial explanations of behavior should not be accepted, and the deeper why of the patient's behavior should always be sought. If he lies, why is it important for him to lie? If he hates, why is it important for him to hate? If he is destructive, why is it important for him to destroy?

Interpersonal relationships, the give-and-take between patient and nurse, are tools of nursing care to be used to promote the patient's health. Upon the skill developed in understanding behavior and its significance will depend much of the ability to use interpersonal relationships as a tool in therapy.

References

Hall, Bernard H.: A colleague looks at psychiatric nursing, Nursing Outlook **2:**66-69, Feb. 1954.

Holmes, Marguerite: The need to be recognized, American Journal of Nursing **61:**86-87, Oct. 1961.

Prange, Arthur J., Jr. and Martin, Harry W.: Aids to understanding patients, American Journal of Nursing **62:**98-100, July 1962.

Schwartz, Morris S. and Shockley, Emmy Lanning: The nurse and the mental patient, New York, 1956, Russell Sage Foundation, pp. 218-230.

Speroff, B. J.: Empathy is important in nursing, Nursing Outlook **4:**326-328, June 1956.

Chapter viii

The nurse and the
individual patient

Regardless of the pattern of behavior that may characterize a patient's mental illness, there are certain general principles that apply to the care of all who show behavior disorders. Everyone has certain basic needs that must be met, no matter how different the surface behavior may be. For example, all of us need a fairly comfortable self-opinion with which to live. One person may attempt to achieve it by striving to excel as an athlete and another as an intellectual. Still another may attempt to bolster his self-opinion by constant criticism of others, making himself seem superior by comparison. Or an individual may imagine himself quite outstanding and retain that opinion by refusing to participate in any experience in which there is the slightest chance that his sterling traits may be challenged. Regardless of the behavior differences, all of these persons are striving to maintain a good opinion of themselves. For this reason, some general principles govern conduct in caring for patients who are ill as persons, no matter what form their illness takes.

Generalizations regarding nursing care must be accompanied by certain cautions. We have no single, generally accepted theory of the cause or cure of mental illness. Therefore, we have no single, solid theoretic basis for psychiatric nursing. The generalizations that follow are guidelines developed through experience and research, and experience underlies the major portion. Such generalizations regarding nursing care might be considered hypotheses. However, nursing care must be provided for patients with psychiatric disorders, and the thoughtful approaches based upon experience and study represent the best we have at the present moment. Psychiatric nursing, in this sense of being based upon a solid and tested theoretic concept, does not differ from nursing in any other clinical area.

Accepting patients exactly as they are

In the ordinary course of events, the average person has certain standards of conduct that he demands of other persons with whom he associates.

Failure to meet those standards on the part of others calls forth retaliatory measures of various degrees. For example, in so simple a matter as eating habits, strong attitudes are typical. The man whose table manners are not impeccable may well expect to be punished for his behavior if he enters social circles in which impeccable table manners are a criterion for social acceptance. He will be ignored, he will be criticized, he may be isolated from group relationships by complete rejection, or he may be openly reprimanded. In any cause, these measures are punitive in nature and are designed to make more or less obvious that certain types of behavior are not acceptable and that acceptance depends upon an alteration or correction of the offensive habit. With a reasonable degree of security and self-confidence, the average person can interpret what is happening and alter his behavior to gain approval and acceptance even though his feelings may be hurt in the process. Most of us are educable and remain so throughout our lives. In addition to correcting behavior in response to the feedback from persons in the environment, the individual with a reasonable degree of security and self-confidence may also be capable of pursuing a course of action he believes to be right despite pressure from others.

When we react with a person who is suffering from an emotional disorder, an entirely different problem is presented. The problem is not one of educating through reason, through the judicious application of approval or disapproval, or through the use of reward and punishment. The patient has already acquired inefficient methods of handling his life problems, and these methods are usually defensive in nature, based on strong emotional needs. Reeducation in deep-seated values and attitudes toward others and the self are the heart of therapy, and this involves a major personality reorganization. The patient needs to unlearn much before he can learn again. He has already been exposed to reason and the use of punishment and reward in society, and such measures have failed. He needs something different, something that gives him an opportunity to see and accept what he must unlearn first before he can bend his energies toward learning again. He needs a very low-pressure social environment in which he can learn to live again with others in much the same manner as a person with paralysis must learn to walk again. A paralyzed patient, newly recovered, is not expected to get out of bed and do a hundred-yard sprint. An emotionally ill patient is not expected to meet normal standards of behavior nor to be punished or rewarded as his behavior approaches or recedes from such standards. He needs, first and foremost, to be accepted as a person exactly as he is.

To accept a patient as a person does not mean we sanction or approve his behavior. We simply acknowledge the fact, by our attitude, that the patient has a right to behave as he does. Conveying acceptance of a patient is not to be confused with resignation or drifting with the situation by the nurse. Acceptance is an active process, a series of positive behaviors designed to convey to the patient a respect for him as an individual human being who possesses worth and dignity as such. Acceptance is expressed through many avenues of approach: nonjudgmental and nonpunitive relationships with the patient, direct and indirect expressions of interest in the patient, recognition and reflection of the patient's feelings, talking with understanding to the patient, listening to the patient, and permitting the patient to express strongly held feelings.

In accepting patients through a nonjudgmental approach, we avoid all moral judgment and its expression—a patient's behavior is no more right or wrong, good or bad, than the pain that accompanies an ulcer is right or wrong. In both instances, symptoms are presented. The danger lies in the fact that the symptoms of a mentally ill patient often occur in an area in which the average person is accustomed to making value or moral judgments. This danger should be faced, and any person working with emotional disorders should be alert to and guard against its appearance in personal feeling about patients. It is not wrong to feel somewhat shocked when a patient is especially crude or vulgar, but it is wrong to make the patient feel that he has offended and must be punished.

A nonpunitive approach to patients means that, although they are

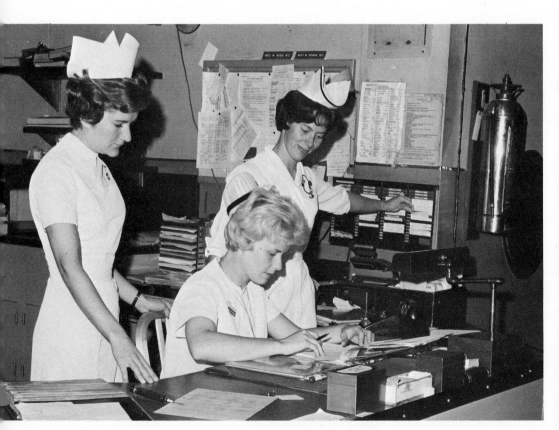

*The familiar cluster pattern of nurses around the desk can be used
to avoid patient contact.*

encouraged to express their feelings and although their behavior may not meet social standards (including one's own), the patient is punished neither directly nor indirectly for his expressions or behavior. The avoidance of retaliation sounds too easy. It is doubtful if a nurse exists who knows she punishes her patients; yet the actual occurrence is quite frequent. To be able to avoid retaliation, a nurse must develop skill in realizing how it can be expressed. The means of punishment are many and varied. They consist of such measures as avoiding a patient except when something must be done for him, telling him something unpleasant for his own good, calling attention to his defects by talking about them, reducing him to a diagnosis, failing to explain what is being done to him, laughing at his fears, being condescending and superior, expecting him to know and behave as though hospital routine were more important than he, demanding that he respect doctors and nurses, and saying the right thing in words but letting the facial expression and body posture convey annoyance and disapproval. There are other means, of course. The point is that the fact that all behavior has meaning and conveys something to others must be accepted. The nurse must study her personal behavior, as well as that of the patient, and the latter is much the easier task.

Another method of accepting patients is to show interest in the patient as a person, not as a case or a clinical problem. The interest shown in reading the patient's chart and in studying textbooks for increased understanding of the development of the behavior pattern is only the first step. Interest in the patient as a person must be shown in the presence of the patient, or where the patient can see evidence of such interest, for it to be brought to the patient's awareness and have any effect on his feelings or behavior. Interest can be shown by seeking out the patient, by using time spent with him on those things in which he is interested, and by awareness of his likes and dislikes. His requests can be met, or the reason for not being able to meet requests can be explained in terms that make sense to him. His comments, complaints, and expressions of approval can be dealt with realistically, not brushed aside. His fears can be accepted as real to him, not treated lightly. Subjects about which he is sensitive can be known and avoided. In other words, there must first be patient-nurse contact that is not always dictated by absolute necessity, and the nurse must be aware of what kind of person the patient is. This knowledge should guide the nurse's behavior so that respect for the patient is there for him to see if and when he is able.

A much neglected method for conveying acceptance to a patient is the simple act of staying with the patient. There are many opportunities for doing this, even if the period of time involved is not long. Staying with a patient seems relatively simple, but it is apparently an art that needs cultivation and is well worth practice.

Acceptance can be conveyed to patients by recognizing the feelings they *do* express. This presents several problems, one of which is that certain segments of our culture place a premium on avoiding the expressions

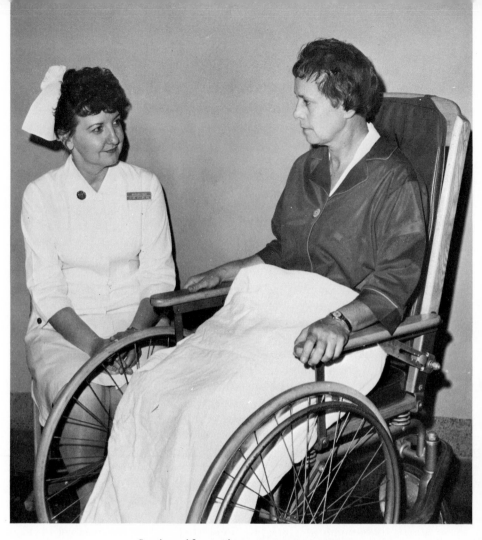

Staying with a patient conveys acceptance.

of strong emotions. Another is the hesitancy on the part of many persons as to what to do when strong emotions are expressed. If one can learn to accept, nonjudgmentally and nonpunititively, the expression of emotions and feelings and then learn to accept one's self as a sounding board for the patient, the first step will be made. One approach that helps in learning to accept the expression of emotions is to focus attention upon understanding what the feeling means to the patient. This requires the development of some degree of skill in identifying the feelings actually expressed. The patient's statement, "I'd like to break someone's neck," means that he is angry. Such expressions are met by the reflection of the *feeling* expressed, not the words. Another method is by an open-end question that leaves the patient free to go in any direction he chooses, that is, it does not direct the patient's answer in any specific direction. Such a question is, "Would you care to tell me about it?" In any case, it is first necessary to practice identifying the feelings expressed by the words patients use. In case of doubt, paraphrasing *what* the patient has said may lead to further patient expression that will clarify the feeling being expressed.

One difficulty in identifying attitudes and feelings may arise because these important emotions may be confused with the intellectual content of the patient's conversation. It is what is revealed concerning feelings that is significant. Most of us can throw up a verbal screen around our emotions, but it can be penetrated by skilled observers who keep asking, "Why? Why? Why?" An example of confusion over content and feeling, their significance, and how they can affect response is given in the following instance. A patient explained that, although he was chairman of his department in a university, he was not trusted by the chancellor. The actual content of this statement would indicate that the patient probably was trusted; otherwise he would not be likely to have held the position he did. A direct response on this basis would be to point that out to the patient. The significant fact in the patient's statement is that *he felt he was not trusted.* This is the feeling expressed.* Practice can develop considerable skill in recognizing feelings and attitudes.

Talking provides a means of conveying acceptance to patients. It can, without doubt, also be misused in the sense that talking can be a means of rejecting patients very effectively. There is an old saying around hospitals that there would be fewer suspicious and critical patients if nurses talked less and listened more. There is some grain of truth in this. In the first place, the nurse should not superimpose her own conversational pattern on the nurse-patient relationship in any situation. The conversation should center on the patient, on his needs and wants, and on his interests, not on the nurse's. In any situation in which the patient's feelings or behavior is predominantly involved, the nurse should learn to analyze her own pattern of verbal responses and learn to use what Porter calls the "understanding" response. This does not mean that this is the only type of response ever to be used by a nurse. When a patient complains of pain that has an organic base, for example, questions that are direct and designed to elicit specific information are necessary. Direct approaches are usually indicated when physical problems or overt problems are present. The more indirect approaches, such as reflection or open-end questions, are more effective when the nursing problems are covert, such as emotional or social problems.

Bernstein, Brophy, McCarthy, and Roepe have classified types of verbal responses as evaluative, hostile, supportive, probing, or understanding. Evaluative responses are those in which the nurse makes a judgment (good or bad) about the patient's feelings and may go on to imply what he ought to feel or do. An example would be a response to a patient's complaint about nursing care in this manner, "Most patients seem to think the nursing care around here is pretty good. You will get better faster if you

---

*Excellent illustrations of how to identify the significant feelings that are expressed by individuals are given by W. U. Snyder and Hildegarde E. Peplau.

have a little more faith in us." Here the nurse implies that the patient is wrong and that he ought to change his attitude for his own sake. Such a response contributes little to patient care. A hostile response is one that rejects the patient through ridicule or blame or denies him the right to have any feelings on the subject at all. An example would be a nurse responding to a patient's complaint about an aide with, "You have no right to complain about her. She's underpaid and overworked, and you take up too much of her time with your constant demands." This type of response can hardly help even an irritated nurse feel better. In the supportive response, based on a misguided conception of what constitutes reassurance, the nurse denies that the patient really has a problem and implies that his concerns or worries are unnecessary. An example would be a nurse telling a patient who has expressed fear about a forthcoming operation that, "Everybody is afraid of operations, but you have a good doctor, and we have a good staff, and everything will be all right." This should accomplish little except to shut off any opportunity for the patient to face and deal with his fear. A probing response is one in which the nurse seeks further information and implies that she has the correct answers, if she only can get enough information. An example would be a nurse who, in response to a patient's complaint that her husband was unfaithful, says, "Let us find out about this. What makes you sure he is?" This probing approach is ineffective in dealing with patient feelings. An understanding response is one in which the nurse tries to understand what the patient is saying from his point of view. An example would be a nurse who replies to a patient's expressed concern over a pending operation with, "You are worried about your operation." This leaves the door open for the patient to explore his feelings further in an atmosphere in which it is safe "to feel." He is "understood." Students need practice to learn how to analyze their own verbal responses, to recognize what they are really saying to patients, and, especially, to develop skill in using the understanding response. Understanding, reflection, and open-end questions are talking skills that convey acceptance to patients.

Listening to patients is another means of conveying acceptance. The art of listening means more than keeping quiet—it includes opening the ears to hear what is said and using the intellect to understand the meaning of what is said. Encouraging patients to do the talking through brief, nondirective comments and through interest in what the patient is saying can be a rewarding experience. Many patients who begin with superficial comments when conversing with a good listener soon get past the superficial stage under the influence of acceptance and will reveal much that is of real significance to them.

Permitting patients to express emotions is another means of expressing acceptance. Patients are overwhelmed by negative emotions and need the opportunity to express such emotions without danger, psychologic or physical, to themselves and others. This principle tends to be in direct contrast to accepted patterns in society. The direct expression of strong

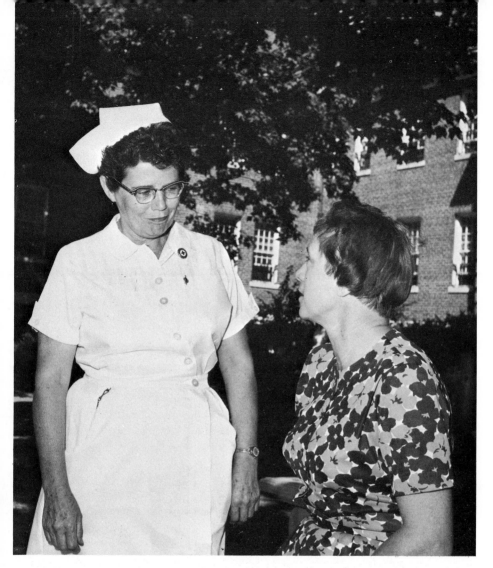

Listening is an active, not a passive, process.

negative emotion tends to call for suppression, and symbolic expression is much better tolerated. It is not exactly safe under normal social conditions to go about striking everyone who is annoying, but it is quite all right to go to a boxing or wrestling match and work off the emotion vicariously. Strong emotions, bottled up and kept out of awareness, are potentially explosive and dangerous. Patients with personality disorders are plagued with negative emotional responses which they have not been able to handle successfully, and these emotions are in need of an outlet. Anxiety, fear, hostility, hatred, and anger should be expected, tolerated, and allowed expression. In fact, the ability of the patient to express a negative emotion is often a very healthy sign. For this reason, the evidences of fear, dislike, and hostility should be encouraged rather than discouraged.

Strange as it may seem, a nurse can sometimes be more help to a psychiatric patient if she is the object of his hostility rather than the object of his affections. Her quiet acceptance of the patient's dislike permits him to discharge an emotion that might otherwise be bottled up, and it also permits the patient to express his negative emotion without the retaliation he expects. One of the real dangers of hatred and hostility to the person who feels them is the fear of retribution they carry. Their expression without punitive return makes it much easier for the patient to learn to be objective about the emotion and to then go on to a more healthy attitude about it in himself.

Vicarious and symbolic methods of releasing negative emotions should be provided until the patient is able to bring his anxiety or hatred out into the open. Metal hammering, punching bags, tennis or badminton, golf, movies, and other activities should be available. It should always be kept in mind, however, that any frank expression of strong negative emotions is healthy for psychiatric patients and that it is most healthy when it is calmly accepted.

If the patient has certain attitudes to unlearn, he must first be able to see them in himself. His behavior is defensive, and any criticism of it strengthens the need for it. Therefore, the patient needs an atmosphere in which his behavior is calmly accepted and no threat is present for him. Only when his behavior is objectively viewed will he be able to view it objectively himself. The first step in helping a patient in the painful process of reeducation is to make him as nondefensive with his illness as possible. Accept him exactly as he is.

Seeking validation from patient

It is the meaning of feelings and behavior *from the patient's point of view* that is of primary importance, and only the patient knows how experience looks to him. Therefore, the logical procedure is to seek validation from the patient to check against the nurse's interpretation of how *he* sees things. If, for example, the nurse's observations lead her to conclude that the patient is avoiding her, she can so state and check with the patient whether her feeling is right or wrong. The matter-of-fact presentation of the nurse's conclusion and the request for validation provide the patient an opportunity to correct or to confirm the conclusion, as only he can do.

Underlying the effectiveness of the process of seeking validation from the patient is one fact upon which all schools of psychiatric thought agree. The essence of the helping relationship is the ability to convey to the patient the sense of trying to understand him and his feelings as they appear to him. Seeking validation conveys this effort.

Orlando[*] reports that patient difficulties arise from misinterpretation and misinformation about a real life situation. Knowing the real situation and knowing the patient frequently do not add up to the correct conclu-

---

[*]Orlando, Ida Jean: The dynamic nurse-patient relationship, New York, 1961, G. P. Putman's Sons.

sions as to what nursing action should be. The nursing element is the meaning of the situation to the patient, and it is the essential step of having the patient validate this meaning that often provides the clue to effective action on the part of the nurse. Effective action is that which relieves distress.

Self-understanding used as a therapeutic tool

In developing skills needed to participate effectively in the care of patients with personality disorders, the nurse must know how to approach realistically the problem of bringing about change within herself. She will become comfortable enough in her relationships with patients to be helpful only when she feels some security about her ability to respond appropriately to patient behavior. The method of approaching this problem is important because it will probably determine how effective the nurse will eventually become. It is not enough to identify the attitude or feeling she *ought* to assume toward specific patients. Knowing how we ought to feel or act does not necessarily change feelings or behavior. In fact, knowing no more than how one ought to feel can produce real feelings of guilt.

It is necessary to be realistic and face the difficulties involved in adjusting the responses of the nurse to patient needs. The behavior of mentally ill patients has a high potential for producing anxiety in the persons who work with them. Anxiety calls forth defenses. It is easy to let one's response to patients be determined by the need to protect one's self from the anxiety aroused. It is perfectly natural to feel anger, resentment, pity, and dislike as well as liking for mentally ill patients. These responses are among those we feel toward people who are not mentally ill. Our first step is to learn as much about behavior as we can so that we can increase our understanding of what is actually happening. This in itself is helpful, but it is not enough. We must apply what we learn to our own behavior and to our own feelings, as well as to those of other persons.

The nurse who feels she ought to be kind and understanding while she is actually feeling irritated with a patient is caught on the horns of a dilemma. The possibility of developing feelings of guilt are good. Feelings are not turned on and off at command. The nurse needs to learn to accept herself as part of learning how to accept others. She can try to identify what she actually feels and thinks as the first step in bringing about change in herself since this will identify what is to be changed. Next she needs to face the fact that simply telling herself not to feel that way is wasted time. The nurse needs to analyze the why's both in her own behavior and in her patient's behavior. It is often helpful to do this with someone else in the situation rather than to try to do it alone. Exchanging experiences frankly with classmates may have some value since it is reassuring to find one's own reactions shared by others. Discussing personal reactions frankly with more experienced persons in the situation is almost a necessity. Participation in group conferences about patient care is another source of help. Such experiences, with increasing knowledge brought to bear on them, contribute to the development of skills in interpersonal relationships

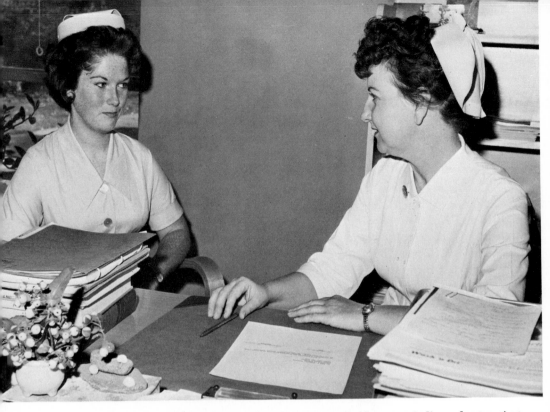

The student nurse's primary resource for discussing her own feelings about patients and nursing is her instructor.

through increased self-understanding and through increased understanding of others.

Orlando* suggests that the nurse discuss frankly with the patient her own reactions to him when those feelings or reactions are a source of difficulty in providing nursing care, as, for example, when the nurse is angered by the patient's behavior. This should be done only if *the nurse gives the patient the reason for her reaction and invites the patient to react.* Such an approach assumes that the nurse first knows why she feels what she feels and can identify correctly her feeling.

Nurse's personal contribution

What each nurse brings to a therapeutic relationship is her own unique contribution—what she is as a person, which is different from what any other person is. This is one of the reasons why there are no standard replies to patient questions, no standard pattern of behavior for any situation in a psychiatric setting. The same words used by two different nurses may well have two different meanings to the same patient. There are no magic words, and stereotyped behavior responses to types of situations are potentially dangerous.

---

*Orlando, Ida Jean: The dynamic nurse-patient relationship, New York, 1961, G. P. Putman's Sons.

It is generally accepted that the consistency of the nurse's feelings and thoughts with her behavior constitute a therapeutic asset. This is why self-understanding of how she really feels is so important. This is why stereo-typed behavior responses to situations and patients is potentially danger-ous. The resulting inconsistency between feelings and actions lessens the nurse's effectiveness in a relationship. This is why the nurse who tries to coax a patient when she would like to swat him is practically never successful. The first problem that needs attention in such a situation is the nurse's own feeling.

The degree of congruence, or consistency in feeling, thoughts, and be-havior, exhibited by the nurse affects her therapeutic potential. The extent to which her behavior reflects what she really is as a unique individual affects her therapeutic potential as well. It is not usually possible to de-velop a helping relationship unless one really wants to, and how the help-ing relationship, if wanted, does develop is an expression of the uniqueness of both the patient and the nurse.

Consistency and patient security

It is axiomatic that all mentally ill patients are insecure and uncertain, no matter what their behavior may appear to be on the surface. Therefore attention to the small and the large details that contribute to security is necessary. One of the most effective measures to promote a sense of se-curity is consistency in experience.

All persons are more comfortable working in a place with which they are familiar than beginning a new job. Not knowing what to expect pro-duces anxiety. Nothing so firmly implants safety in expectation as con-sistent experience. And consistency in all areas of experience is valuable to the psychiatric patient, for it builds in his environment something upon which he can depend.

The use of consistency is of value in routine, in attitudes, and in de-fining the limitations placed upon the patient. A routine in a psychiatric hospital that is fairly consistent helps the patient by reducing the number of decisions he is called upon to make and by giving him something upon which he can depend.

Consistency in the attitude of personnel toward him is profoundly important to the patient. Generally speaking, other people are not an ex-pected source of comfort and consolation to the psychiatric patient. It helps him if he learns through day-by-day contact exactly what he can expect. It is even more helpful if he is constantly and continuously exposed to an atmosphere of quiet acceptance. There is nothing particularly unusual about this since people are more comfortable with someone who is on all occasions friendly and yet not disturbed by faults. Occasional lapses will be excused but not enjoyed. Consistency in attitude on the part of the in-dividual members of personnel is important, but consistency from person to person and shift to shift should be deliberately planned. The necessity for teamwork is quite obvious.

Although the acceptance of patient behavior and the permissive therapeutic atmosphere have been stressed, the permissiveness is limited. Patients cannot be allowed to do exactly as they please for rather obvious reasons. The homicidal patient is not permitted to kill others; the suicidal patient is not permitted to kill himself; the overactive patient is not permitted to completely exhaust himself; nor is the suspicious patient permitted to starve himself. That the patient *feels* that way is accepted, that the patient has a right to feel that way is accepted, but limitations are drawn beyond which his behavior is not allowed to go. The definition of limits and their enforcement are tasks that require a great deal of tact and understanding since the potential psychologic threat to the patient can be handled in such a way as to place him on the defensive in his relationships with personnel. Consistency in quiet, matter-of-fact enforcement of limitations is one of the most effective methods of using the limits as a contribution to the patient's security. They must be something upon which the patient can rely. The attempt to win a patient's liking by being more permissive with him than other members of personnel is disastrous for the patient; whereas it may earn his personal liking, even though this is doubtful, it contributes to his confusion and insecurity. Actual limitations on a patient's behavior should be determined by the team under the direction of the physician, and those limitations should be *consistently* enforced by everyone who comes in contact with the patient.

Reassurance

All of us need reassurance at one time or another, and psychiatric patients need it constantly. However, here again we come upon the fact that it is profoundly important to understand the meaning of experience to the patient, rather than to act upon the premise of how *we* would feel in the same circumstances. One of the most reassuring experiences for a patient is the professional competence of the nurse. In the care of emotionally maladjusted patients, a large measure of the nurse's competence will depend on her ability to see how situations appear to the patient. Reassurance is a great deal more subtle than telling the patient that he will get well, that his fears are groundless, that he is a nice person, and that all will end well.

Verbal reassurance is effective only when it does not contradict a false concept the patient needs. The patient, punishing himself with the firm idea that he will die at midnight, is not likely to be very receptive to reassurance that he will be alive and healthy when the nurse comes on duty the next day. The patient who is sure he is crippled for life by heart disease is not likely to be made very happy by the assurance that there is nothing wrong with his heart. Instead, he will probably cling more strongly to his belief. The value of the idea to the patient and his emotional need for it should be carefully assessed before it is used as a point for verbal reassurance.

Reassurance can best be given the patient by interest in him as a person, by attention to matters that are important to him, and by allowing him to be as sick as he needs to be. It can be given through awareness and acceptance of how the patient really feels. Reassurance is also given by doing all these things without asking anything of the patient in return, such as improved behavior or a show of appreciation.

Change in patient behavior through emotional experience

The major focus in psychiatric therapy and in psychiatric nursing is upon the feeling aspect of the personality, not upon the intellectual aspects. One of the more difficult problems for nurses in working with mentally ill patients is a problem that they tend to have with difficult patients in any field of nursing. The problem centers in the naive faith of most of us that change in behavior is easily produced by the use of reason. If we tell a patient what he ought to do and why he ought to do it, we expect him to change his way because "he knows better." We then wash our hands of any further responsibility. The frequency with which nurses are disappointed in this expectation is sufficient proof that *telling people* is not an effective method of changing behavior. This is especially true when the patient has emotional difficulties.

If a patient could be reasoned out of his psychotic ideas, he would never need treatment in a hospital. He would simply need to sit down with some very bright soul who would point out the fallacies in the patient's thinking, and all would be well. The patient's pattern of behavior has been developed to defend himself from anxiety-producing stress, and in building the defensive pattern, reason has been used as one of the tools to support the psychotic or neurotic structure. The patient cannot, therefore, be reasoned into a better state of adjustment.

Any attempt to reason anyone out of a belief based on strong emotional needs is doomed, no matter how well adjusted the person may be. Although it is true that false beliefs based on the inadequate or inaccurate information can be changed when the correct information is made available, this does not apply to false beliefs that have a strong emotional component.

All of us have our blind spots in which a cherished belief overrules all facts and all reason. The more such beliefs are challenged, the more vigorously are they defended. Knowledge and reason are not panaceas for the cure of emotional problems. Corrective *emotional* experience, however, can bring about behavior changes in such situations.

Any effort to use intellect and reason in dealing with patient's ideas that have a strong emotional component must be avoided. From the outside looking in, it sometimes seems as though the patient simply *must* be able to see the reason for his behavior and correct it. This is from the outside—it is necessary to try to see it from the inside. The patient's emotional need for his beliefs will resist any intellectual challenge brought by others. Reason is not an effective weapon in changing patient behavior.

Unless given specific directions to the contrary, the interpretation of his behavior to a patient should be avoided. By interpretation is meant telling the patient about the meaning of his behavior or explaining his unconscious motivations. The ideal goal of therapy is to help the patient to such a degree of emotional security that he can develop and use an understanding of his behavior. Such understanding cannot be forced upon him from outside. Nor can he use his knowledge until he can emotionally accept it.

Insight, or the understanding of one's own motivation and behavior, can be an extremely painful experience. Its development in a patient with an emotional disorder must necessarily be slow and support must be present to enable him to tolerate the knowledge that his behavior is not always altruistically motivated. Interpretation can be done only when the patient is ready for it, secure enough to tolerate it, and able to apply it to alter his behavior. It is useless in terms of improvement before the patient is ready for it, and the only thing it can accomplish under such circumstances is to increase the pressure on the patient and make him feel more uncomfortable. Therefore, interpretation of behavior is to be avoided.

In this connection, it is helpful to remember that attitudes the patient himself does not recognize should not be identified for him. If he were able to tolerate such attitudes in himself, he would then be likely to identify them himself. By way of example, a patient may criticize the hospital personnel sharply, calling them incompetent and a disgrace to the profession they represent. Along with information gained from previous observation, the nurse may be fully aware that the patient is showing an attitude of rebellion toward authority. This the patient has not expressed, but he has expressed an attitude of contempt toward personnel. To reflect the latter is acceptable since the patient has said it; to reflect the rebellion toward authority, revealed indirectly, would be a threat to the patient. He has not recognized and accepted his feeling toward authority as part of himself. Insight can be a threat or a help, depending on the course of the patient's illness, and its danger as well as its value should be kept in mind.

Avoiding increased patient anxiety

As a general rule, fear and anxiety are already problems with which the patient has been unable to cope. Careful study of situations, topics, or approaches that seem to indicate a resultant increase in anxiety in the patient should be made. The knowledge gained should be used to contribute to the patient's comfort.

Certain general types of situations can be avoided since an increase in anxiety can almost safely be predicted if the situation arises. Direct contradiction of psychotic ideas is almost certain to produce anxiety in patients since such ideas are always based on deep emotional needs. The effect is approximately the same as threatening to take crutches away from a person who cannot walk without them. Demands upon the patient that he obviously cannot meet are also certain anxiety producers. To insist that a depressed patient cheer up, that an overactive patient go sit down and be quiet, or that a withdrawn patient initiate and carry through group activities simply places the patient in the position of having failed again. Failure causes anxiety in persons already insecure. The level of activity required of the patient should be adjusted with regard to the limitations his symptoms place on him.

The indiscriminate use of medical and psychiatric terminology in front of patients can often produce anxiety. Such terminology identifies a person as a member of a select group and shuts out those who do not belong. It is a thoughtless rejection of patients. In the same sense, careless conversation where patients can overhear may produce anxiety.

No attention should ever be called to a patient's defects, failing abilities, peculiarities, or failure. If a patient wishes to mention them, accept them calmly and without criticism. To focus attention on weaknesses increases anxiety. In any personal relationships it is a wise rule to concentrate on the individual's strengths.

Insincerity can also produce anxiety since it leaves the patient uneasy as to what to expect and uncertain as to where he stands. Since patients tend to integrate those elements of experience which confirm their poor opinion of themselves, they are most likely to interpret obvious insincerity as an attempt to conceal an unpleasant opinion of themselves.

The initial experience in the hospital, with its differences and its newness, is fraught with anxiety-producing potentials. Careful orientation to the hospital, explanation and preparation for what is about to happen, and a sensitivity for how the patient feels about his admission are necessary. The initial emotional experience of admission can influence the patient's attitude toward the hospital for a long time to come. Treatment begins with the admission procedure.

Threats, sharp commands, and indifference to a patient's reactions have no place in the care of psychiatric patients or in the care of any patients, for that matter. Threats, sharp commands, and indifference cause anxiety.

In ordinary social relationships, family, friends, home, and occupation are frequent sources of conversational feelers used to bridge the initial gap between not knowing and knowing other people. In working with psychiatric patients, we find again a contrast to usual social practice. Questions about family, friends, home, and job are not very good areas for conversational efforts during the exploratory stages of establishing relationships with patients. The source of the patient's difficulties may arise from and are always related to his interrelationships with those who are closest to him. Feelings of hostility for family members may be the source of a patient's feelings of guilt, and conversation in which the patient admits his hostility may cause anxiety. In regard to family and their members, occupations, and likes and dislikes, always listen when a patient talks, but be careful to avoid judgments or comments that may add to a patient's anxiety. All of these are touchy subjects and should be carefully handled. Generally speaking, it is a good rule to follow the patient's lead in selecting areas of conversation, at least until one knows the patient.

When a patient does burst forth with a confession of some feeling or experience about which he obviously feels strongly, care must be exercised not to presume on the revelation. The patient should be treated exactly as he was previously, and mention of what was revealed should come first from the patient. If he seems standoffish or sarcastic, it should be realized that he may be regretting what he has said. The same relationship should be held open for him until he can accept it again, and the incident, including the patient's reaction to it, should be brought up only by the patient.

Observation of reason for behavior

Everything the patient says and does should be observed, recorded, and reported for the information of those directing the patient's therapeutic program. In addition, for her own information in planning the patient's care, the nurse should learn to recognize the attitudes expressed by the patient, the attitudes he does not recognize in himself, and the attitudes he has toward himself. The patient's behavior should be analyzed to seek its motivation and to understand what the patient is attempting to accomplish. The observation of patient behavior should contribute to the understanding that is basic to good care.

One way to improve skill in understanding why the patient behaves as he does is continuous practice in predicting patient behavior in certain situations. Of course, it is helpful first to learn as much about a patient as possible and, armed with understanding of the patient's basic problems, then make an intelligent guess as to what he will do. When the prediction is right, analyze why it was right and consider what other action the patient might reasonably have taken. When the prediction is wrong, analyze why it was wrong and seek the logical reason for the patient's actual behavior. In any instance of patient behavior, seek answers to the following questions. What is the goal of the behavior? Why did the patient behave as he did?

Understanding why patients behave as they do is much easier if the nurse can view behavior objectively. Objectivity is the ability to evaluate a situation, in this case the patient's behavior, on the basis of what is actually happening, rather than on the basis of one's personal feelings. Complete objectivity would be possible only in a vacuum. Reasonable objectivity is capable of being reached and is a practical goal.

There are several things that objectivity is not—it is not coldness, indifference, or absence of feeling. It is rather the ability to not let one's judgment be confused by the presence of warmth or resentment when the patient is concerned. Emotionally reached conclusions can be detrimental to the patient's welfare.

In order to be objective it is necessary to indulge, to some extent at least, in introspection in order to recognize one's own feelings and guard against their influence on judgment. A real danger, and one hard to detect, is the exploitation of patients to meet the nurse's own emotional needs. Nurses are human beings, too, and they need to be liked, to be respected as persons, and to be important to others. They need recognition, appreciation, and reassurance. However, they are expected to meet these emotional needs other than through patients. With mentally ill patients, the nurse must be prepared to give and to expect no return other than the pleasure of seeing patients recover. Above all, the nurse must lead a balanced life and have genuine sources of emotional satisfaction other than her patients. Whenever she finds herself being critical of patients, defending or justifying herself, demanding that patients treat her in a certain manner, or evaluating patient's behavior in terms of right or wrong, the nurse is then in danger of letting her own emotional needs take precedence over those of patients. Working with psychiatric patients requires a certain hard-headed and frequently painful honesty. The ability to accept the faults one cannot change and the personal limitations within herself are as important for the nurse as her ability to accept patients. One is difficult without the other.

Realistic nurse-patient relationship

It is essential that the relationship the nurse offers the patient be founded on a realistic basis. Much as one might like to be all things to all people or all things to some people, it is hardly possible in any situation. The professional relationship of nurse and patient, warm and understanding, can help greatly in establishing the kind of environment patients need to give them an opportunity to get well. Limitations within the relationship can be drawn, and, unconventional as psychiatric nursing may be at times, the limitations that characterize professional relationships can be a genuine relief. A person must crawl before he walks, and the patient can begin with a relationship that crawls in the sense that its demands on him are few and that he is not expected to live up to the demands of closer and more intimate situations. In addition, a professional relationship protects the patient from demanding more than he can possibly receive and feeling betrayed as a consequence. What one has a right to expect from a close friend is more in some respects than one can expect from a nurse, no matter how friendly she may be. The professional basis of the relationship is a support to the patient.

In addition, the nurse should understand and function with the understanding that the nurse-patient relationship is a dynamic one. It has a beginning, it develops once a relationship is established, and it has an end. The key to other aspects of a relationship lies in the initial phase when it is being established, for this determines the direction of other aspects. A relationship based on mutual respect and trust will tolerate mistakes and the strains and stresses of termination.

References

Bernstein, Lewis, Brophy, Mary, McCarthy, Mary Jane, and Roepe, Ruby: Teaching nurse-patient relationships; An experimental study, Nursing Research 3:80-84, Oct. 1954.

Brill, Norman Q.: The importance of understanding yourself, American Journal of Nursing 57:1325-1326, Oct. 1957.

Burd, Shirley F., and Marshall, Margaret A.: editors, Some clinical approaches to psychiatric nursing, New York, 1963, Macmillan Co.

Connolly, Mary Grace: What acceptance means to patients, American Journal of Nursing 60:1754-1757, Dec. 1960.

Eldred, Stanley H.: Improving nurse-patient communication, American Journal of Nursing 60:1600-1602, Nov. 1960.

Gregg, Dorothy: Reassurance, American Journal of Nursing 55:171-174, Feb. 1955.

Hale, Shirley L., and Richardson, Julia H.: Terminating the nurse-patient relationship, American Journal of Nursing 63:116-119, Sept. 1963.

Hays, Joyce Samhammer: Focusing on feelings, Nursing Outlook 10:332-333, May 1962.

Hewitt, Helon, and Pesznecker, Betty L.: Blocks to communicating with patients, American Journal of Nursing 64:101-103, July 1964.

Hyde, Robert M., and Coggan, Catherine M.: When nurses have guilt feelings, American Journal of Nursing 58:233-236, Feb. 1958.

Knowles, Lois N.: How can we reassure patients? American Journal of Nursing 59:834-835, June 1959.

Leib, Eloise: A student looks at the psychosocial aspects of patient care, Nursing Outlook 10:799-800, Dec. 1962.

Lewis, Garland K. and Holmes, Marguerite J.: Meddling with emotions, Nursing Outlook 9:405-407, July 1961.

Litwack, Janice, and Litwack, Lawrence: Four stages of nursing care, American Journal of Nursing 62:95-96, Jan. 1962.

Maloney, Elizabeth: Does the psychiatric nurse have independent functions? American Journal of Nursing 62:61-63, June 1962.

Orlando, Ida Jean: The dynamic nurse-patient relationship, New York, 1961, G. P. Putnam's Sons.

Peplau, Hildegard E.: Interpersonal techniques; The crux of psychiatric nursing, American Journal of Nursing 62:50-54, June 1962.

Peplau, Hildegard E.: Interpersonal relations in nursing, New York, 1952, G. P. Putnam's Sons, pp. 17-42, 263-309.

Peplau, Hildegard E.: Talking with patients, American Journal of Nursing 60:964-966, July 1960.

Porter, E. H., Jr.: An introduction to therapeutic counseling, New York, 1950, Houghton Mifflin Co.

Rogers, Carl R.: A counseling approach to human problems, American Journal of Nursing 56:994-997, Aug. 1956.

Rogers, Carl R.: Client-centered therapy, New York, 1951, Houghton Mifflin Co.

Sawatzky, Gordon and Hardin, Harry T.: Making the most of the patient's ego assets, Nursing Outlook 9:694-696, Nov. 1961.

Schwartz, Morris S., and Shockley, Emmy Lanning: The nurse and the mental patient, New York, 1956, Russell Sage Foundation, pp. 218-230.

Snyder, William U.: Case-book of non-directive counseling, New York, 1947, Houghton Mifflin Co.

Travelbee, Joyce: What do we mean by rapport? American Journal of Nursing 63:70-72, Feb. 1963.

Chapter ix

The nurse in the
social setting

In recent years there has been an increasing realization of the importance of the social structure of the hospital and ward units upon the progress of therapeutic efforts for mentally ill patients. Until recently, mental hospitals have been built, organized, and operated on the basis of providing minimal physical hygiene, control, and custodial care. The physical setup and the organization of patient care are suspected of contributing in no small degree to patient tendencies to relinquish responsibility for themselves and to regress in behavior. Hospitals themselves have probably made a substantial contribution to the increase in the number of patients on the "back wards."

The hospital setting has operated to convey considerably less than respect for the worth of the individual admitted as a patient. In most situations, personal clothing is removed and replaced by a somewhat unattractive, regimented garb. Little is expected of the patient by way of responsibility for his own behavior since most decisions are made for him. He is placed on a rigid institutional routine that gets certain kinds of work done, but pays little heed to the patient's own needs, desires, or accustomed behavior. He lives in a drab, institutional setting. If he is "good," he is permitted to participate in menial tasks or busy work. If he works hard and cooperates with the staff, he may come to occupy a favored status on the unit where he lives. He may even become one of the two-column regiments that shuffle each day to the laundry, the farm, or some other detail and then shuffle back each evening, after a routine day's work to a large, impersonal dormitory. The grinding operation of the institution wears down his already damaged sense of worth and dignity slowly but surely.

Hospitals of the very recent past, and to some extent present-day hospitals, also offered an unrealistic social setting. Patients become ill in their relationships with other people in everyday life in the social sphere in which they live. If they are to become well, part of the process will certainly consist of learning how to refunction effectively in the social world from which they come. By and large, in its social structure the hospital bears little relationship to the realities of everyday life outside its walls. To learn to adjust well to its values, routines, and program of activities gives the patient little preparation for a return home.

Recent developments in social therapy

Increased awareness of the importance of factors such as those indicated in the previous paragraphs has led to varied attempts to restructure the social organization of the hospital and its units along lines more consistent with principles of therapy. Among these efforts have been such measures as patient self-government, patient participation in the health team that plans his therapy, total-push therapy, habit training, group therapy, open-door policy, home care programs, day-care or night-care centers, halfway houses, and extended mental hygiene clinics. Such efforts, combined with advances in chemotherapy and increased public understanding of mental illness, have led to decreases in the number of patients hospitalized in some states although the number of admissions has not decreased. What appears to be occurring is not a real decrease in the incidence of mental illness, but a shift in the locale where patients are being treated. When increased social treatment has been accepted as part of therapy, there has also been a trend for patients who are not discharged to improve to an extent that they can be placed on better hospital units and participate more productivity in institutional life. One of the hopeful aspects of the effective use of the social environment is that it has not led to any great need for an increase in personnel. The more effective use of available personnel has produced some amazing results.

The use of a social approach to psychiatric therapy is not new. An outstanding example is the town of Gheel in Belgium, which has provided community care for mentally ill persons since the Middle Ages. Here approximately 2,500 patients are cared for in homes in the community, where the patients participate in the life of the families with whom they are placed. They have meaningful responsibilities, as well as privileges, in such home life. Although seen by physicians only about once a month, they are visited frequently by district nurses who learn to know them well and who are in a position to seek the help of a physician when it is indicated. Patients do not lose social status completely, but are treated as persons with limitations much as any other handicapped group. They are respected as individuals and assume considerable responsibility for themselves, something that would arouse consternation in less progressive mental institutions. An important aspect of the attitude toward mental illness and mentally ill patients is revealed by the fact that personnel and families in Gheel feel that every patient can be placed in a home that will be helpful to him, even though it may require four, five, or more placements before the right family is found. The feeling that a patient, regardless of his condition, can be helped is an essential component of care.

The resurgence of interest in using the social environment therapeutically has led to considerable experimentation, and results have ranged from good to amazing when the experimentation was carried out with adequate preparation, planning, and administrative support. Among psychiatric hospitals that have been working with a team approach that includes psychiatrists, nurses, aides, and departments such as occupational therapy and social service, some hospitals have included the patient on the team, with good results. The patient participates in the exploration of his treatment needs and his planned therapy. This more democratic approach to therapy conveys to the patient a respect for his rights as an individual and the acknowledgement of at least some degree of responsibility for himself.

Some hospitals have used patient self-government as an aid in therapy. Patients determine and enforce, to varying degrees in varying hospitals, the rules and regulations under which they live. On the whole, such participation in control of their environment has been considered an effective means of encouraging patients to take an active part in their therapy, emphasizing as it does their potential for constructive social action.

A technique increasingly used throughout the country is the "ward meeting" of patients and personnel to discuss frankly and jointly, with equal responsibility for solution, the problems of daily living encountered in the patient care unit. The regularity and consistency of such meetings affect their value. They are most commonly held weekly, although timing varies from institution to institution. Both staff and patients must face honestly the effect they have on others, and the staff has an opportunity to provide patients with a healthy model for handling anxiety-arousing experiences. Such meetings also provide a good reality-testing situation. Patient-staff meetings are not new by any means, but their more extensive use is new.

An organization of the pattern of unit operation, based upon the improvement of patient behavior, has been tried with patients on many levels of adjustment. Depending upon the level of patient behavior when the reorganization is undertaken, several patterns have emerged. At the lowest level is the habit-training program designed to improve patient habits in regard to basic behavior. This includes such factors as toilet training, eating habits, personal hygiene, and personal appearance. Patients who are past this stage are placed on more active programs which include a planned schedule of activities that heavily involves not only the nursing department, but also departments such as occupational therapy, recreational therapy, group therapy, phychology, and others. This is sometimes called a total-push program. Other hospitals have organized units designed primarily to promote social interaction among patients and among patients and staff. Experiments with this type of approach have pointed out that the potential ability of patients to respond is frequently vastly underrated. Also underrated is the potential therapeutic contribution of personnel. Characteristic of successful experimentation in these areas has been the provision of group sessions for all personnel involved in patient care, in which their problems and feelings can be explored.

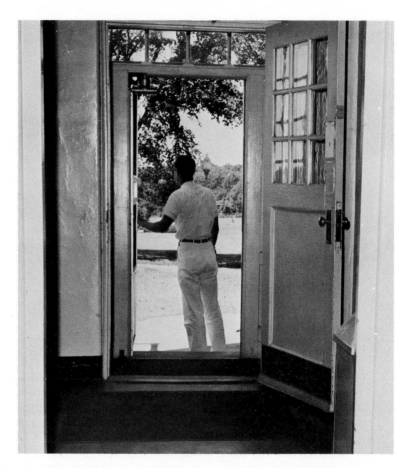

The open door symbolizes the resurgence of a nonrestraint philosophy in the care of mentally ill patients.

Another increase in services for mentally ill patients has been the expanding use of group therapy sessions. Such therapy is being provided by psychiatrists, psychologists, guidance personnel, and nurses, among others. Since at the present time nurses require preparation beyond the basic curriculum for this activity, discussion of this is limited. This constitutes a potential role for the staff nurse in psychiatric nursing for the future, however.

Another movement, which has progressed somewhat further in Great Britain than in America, is the open-door policy. Interpretation of this movement has ranged all the way from changing little except opening locked doors to institutions in which patients and staff participate freely and equally on their respective levels of ability in patient treatment. Perhaps the outstanding example of the latter is Belmont Hospital in England where patients share in all of the important functions of the hospital, where staff and patients are under obligation to help each other, and where nothing is sacred since patients and staff may be held accountable for anything they do in the hospital or outside of it. The staff gives up its authoritarian role and symbols. Daily community meetings are a major aspect of the short, intensive treatment provided, and every one in the hospital participates. Patients show remarkable ability to develop insight into their problems. Here again patients are respected, and they carry responsibility for their own behavior.

One of the more hopeful aspects of recent developments is the recognition of the need to bring the hospital and its patients closer to the community and to develop supplementary means of treatment that keep patients more closely in touch with realistic social settings. Home care or the placement of patients in foster homes is being used to a greater extent. Follow-up care by hospital staffs or by public health agencies, combined with more careful preparation for the patient's return home, is being provided in greater measure. In some institutions, family group sessions are offered to the relatives of a patient during his hospitalization as part of the therapeutic plan. Some hospitals are providing day and/or night centers where patients spend part of the day in the hospital and the rest of it in the community. Psychiatric units for care of mentally ill patients are more often part of a general hospital. In addition, mental hygiene clinic services are increasing.

In all of these movements there are certain common elements that may be major factors in their therapeutic results. First, all are based on a more clear-cut expression, by the use of social environment, of respect for the individual patient as a person of worth and dignity. Second, all express genuine expectation that the patient can improve. Third, all reduce the social distance between patients and staff. Fourth, all provide a more realistic social setting for therapy. Fifth, all emphasize and provide meaningful tasks for patients.

Three rather clear-cut trends are apparent in these recent developments. One is the impact of higher expectations of patient behavior on the part of personnel—as nurses and others expect patient improvement, it occurs. Thus the use of personnel attitudes toward changed patient behavior is recognized as a therapeutic tool. A second trend is the recognition and use of the value system of the social setting in which patients are treated. The implicit as well as the explicit goals of patients and staff have their impact on the extent to which the environment is actually therapeutic. The study of such goals and values and the resulting change, if needed and if possible, also constitute therapeutic tools. A third trend is the greater emphasis upon how personnel handle their own problems and meet their own needs and the impact of this upon patient therapy. Undoubtedly, there is an increasing emphasis upon staff ability to openly express and explore their feelings, not only among themselves but with patients as well. The old traditional pattern of repressing emotional responses and denying their existence is under fire from all sides. Emotional honesty and growing emotional maturity are pretty well considered musts for nurses as well as for others, not only in the care of mentally ill patients, but in the care of all patients.

Principles of nursing care

No definite, concrete directions as to how a nurse can most effectively function in the group setting of the hospital unit, the mental hygiene clinic, or other social setting can yet be postulated with supreme conviction. However, there seems some reason to believe that certain generalizations might at least be helpful guides for testing in action at the present time. The following principles are offered in this spirit.

It might also be wise to keep in mind that social therapy, to be effective, requires attitudes and activities from others than nurses. Without administrative support, without the active participation of medical and allied groups, and without active assistance by aides and others involved in patient care, the nurse may well be faced with frustration. However, it might also be noted that in practically all of the successful experiments in social therapy somewhere there has been a prime mover who instigated change and carried it through with the help of others.

Democratic group setting consistent with therapeutic goals. A group that functions under democratic processes rather than under authoritarian imposition is a group that holds thereapeutic possibilities. Such a group recognizes individual worth and responsibility; yet it does not demand that the individual produce more than he is capable of doing. To the extent that the patient is able, it does permit his participation in decisions affecting him and in carrying out those decisions.

Democracy is not mob rule. Authority exists in a democratic situation, but it resides in competency that is accepted by the group. Perhaps the greatest distinction between democratic and authoritarian approaches lies in the use of authority by each. In the authoritation approach, it is used to impose decisions, to manipulate people, and to control situations in the interest of the authority figure. In the democratic approach, authority is used to forward the goals of the group. When mentally ill patients are in a democratic setting, the goals of such a group must necessarily be improvement of patients' health status. Since this can hardly be achieved by any except patients, their participation in and commitment to this goal is imperative. Democratic processes foster such group orientation; authoritarian processes tend to negate it.

Therapeutic group characterized by permissiveness. A permissive group atmosphere is one in which patients are free to express and to explore their feelings. Such a group is feeling oriented rather than intellectually oriented. Patients are neither judged nor punished for expressed feelings, nor for what they do or have done. A premium is placed upon facing emotional problems, rather than upon accomplishing things. This does not mean that patients are not brought face to face with the reaction of other patients to their behavior or expressions, but that the members of the group learn to focus upon understanding themselves and others, rather than upon judging and punishing each other.

A permissive atmosphere is one in which the patient is free to be himself. It includes respect for his limitations and for those abilities not limited by his illness. He is encouraged to assume all the responsibilities for himself that he can, and he is not required to assume responsibilities that he cannot handle.

Limitations within the group setting are clearly drawn and consistently enforced. These limitations are preferably set by the group within which the patient functions, including staff and patients, and all members of the group are responsible for the enforcement of limitations. Patients frequently show good insight into their own and other patients' behavior and can contribute much to defining and setting limitations. When group assets are used, however, the current level of behavior of the group must be the basis for approach. A unit of extremely regressed patients should be activated with limited goals, such as basic habit training for an immediate project. As patients improve, group goals can be raised.

Socialization and patient interaction with others supported and encouraged. The activity pattern of a ward unit should be organized to promote activities that encourage patient interaction with other patients and with staff. Activities that permit patients to function in isolated fashion without committing themselves in any personal or meaningful way to an activity are of doubtful value except as busy work. Tasks that can be carried out with others—that involve interpersonal contacts, joint decisions, joint planning, and joint activity—promote interaction. Such activities, particularly in a permissive setting, provide patients with an opportunity to explore their social skills and to improve them. The unit that allows or encourages patients to withdraw into themselves encourages regression.

If, for patients who tend to withdraw, the staff will continually reach toward them and allow them plenty of time to respond, personnel will forcibly realize that all too often the patient's ability to respond is vastly underestimated. Patients are aware of much that personnel do not recognize. They learn the pattern of behavior and the predominate social values of the setting in which they are placed and adapt themselves accordingly. If they are placed in a unit with one of its primary goals the interaction of the patients with others, the tendency to regress can often be reversed.

Therapeutic effect enhanced by close social relationship between staff and patients. The social distance between staff and patients in the traditional mental institution is a wide gulf. Most of the new social approaches to the treatment of patients have brought staff and patients more closely together, and they share meaningful tasks and participate in the life of the institution they share. In fact, there is some speculation that the factor that has produced results in patient improvement is related to this lessened social distance. Staff who become participants with patients, rather than observers or control agents, apparently affect positively the course of the illness of patients.

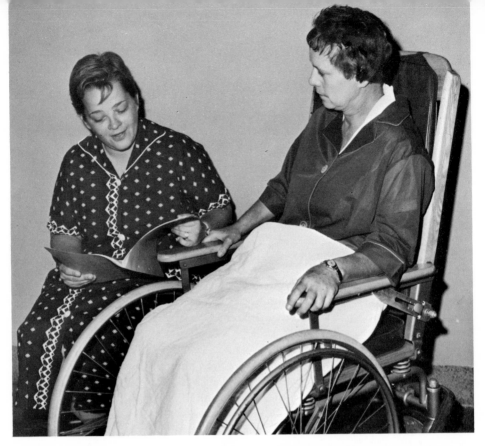

Patients can help each other with benefit to all.

Actually, there exists a very close relationship between the interest and the involvement of staff and the participation of patients. There also exists a very close relationship between good therapeutic results and patient participation. It follows, therefore, that staff interest and personal involvement with patients has a genuine therapeutic effect.

Patients help themselves and each other. Given the opportunity, patients can help themselves get well. To a great extent, this has to do with the attitude of personnel who work with patients. Once this fact is accepted, it can then be carried into action. When the staff believes this, it becomes possible to offer patients such opportunities by respect for them as individuals and by permitting them to take an active part in their own therapy.

When patients are given an opportunity to help other patients, they are experiencing responsibility and satisfaction in a task that holds real meaning. There has been much discussion about the extent to which patients have helped each other get well. In some instances, recovered patients have testified that relationships with particular patients have been extremely helpful to them. In some of the more progressive hospitals, patients have definite assignments that include responsibility for the care of other patients. Such assignments range from responsibility for toileting a regressed patient to instructing groups of patients in a skill. Such assignments and responsibilities for others have been demonstrated to be effective when the patient's ability to contribute has been carefully assessed and when the staff attitude toward the assigned task is positive.

Group approach more effective first with patients who respond positively. When the nurse desires to approach a group with a suggestion or a question, it is usually more effective to direct the question or suggestion to a specific patient whom she can reasonably expect to respond in a positive fashion. The pressure to conform, or not to disagree, which has infiltrated our society has also extended its influence into our hospitals, which reflect the society of which they are a part. Such an approach encourages others who are positively inclined to express themselves and brings some group pressure to support the desired outcome.

Social setting as realistic as patient limitations allow. The social organization of the therapeutic institution should not be at complete variance with the background from which patients come. If it is, it can offer the patient little in better social adjustment and better social relationships on which to build in preparation for return to the community. This means, in a general sense, that the institution should respect the rights of individuals, should be democratic in orientation, should allow for individual difference, and should value behaviors that are socially constructive.

In effect, it means that hospital organization, routines, and activities support and encourage the kind of patient behavior that will be helpful to him when he returns to society.

Nurse's activities coordinated with all groups participating in patient care. This principle is so obvious that it requires no explanation. When there is group participation in social therapy, the activities of all who have part in the social situation must be coordinated in order to assure that the desired therapeutic goals are shared and implemented by all.

References

Bennett, Leland R.: A therapeutic community, Nursing Outlook 9:423-425, July 1961.

Briggs, Dennie Lyon: Social psychiatry in Great Britain, American Journal of Nursing 59:215-220, Feb. 1959.

Briggs, Denniel and Wardell, Marion F.: A locked ward was opened, American Journal of Nursing 61:102-105, Sept. 1961.

Brown, Esther Lucile: Newer dimensions of patient care. Part I. The use of the physical and social environment of the general hospital for therapeutic purposes, New York, 1961, Russell Sage Foundation.

Brown, Esther Lucile: Newer dimensions of patient care. Part II. Improving staff motivation and competence in the general hospital, New York, 1962, Russell Sage Foundation.

Brown, Esther Lucile: Newer dimensions of patient care. Part III. Patients as people, New York, 1964, Russell Sage Foundation.

Bueker, Kathleen and Warrick, Annette: Can nurses be group therapists, American Journal of Nursing 64:114-116, May 1964.

Burke, Nancy: Therapy—eight hours a day. In The nurse and groups of patients or clients, New York, American Nurses Association, 1962.

Carleton, Estelle I. and Johnson, Joan Canatsy: A therapeutic milieu for borderline patients, American Journal of Nursing 61:64-67, Jan. 1961.

Chamberlain, Amparo S.: Visit to Gheel, American Journal of Nursing 59:68-70, Jan. 1959.

Christman, Luther: Interpersonally speaking, Nursing Forum 1:109-125, 1962.

Findley, Annie P.: They're learning to live again, American Journal of Nursing 61:84-86, June 1961.

Fleming, Richard, Grayson, David M., and McLanahan, Winifred: An after-care program for patients discharged from mental hospitals, Nursing Outlook 9:545-547, Sept. 1961.

Greenblatt, Milton, York, Richard H., and Brown, Esther Lucile: From custodial to therapeutic patient care in mental hospitals, New York, 1955, Russell Sage Foundation.

Hays, Joyce Samhammer: The psychiatric nurse as sociotherapist, American Journal of Nursing 62:64-67, June 1962.

Holmes, Marguerite, Lefley, Doris, and Werner, Jean A.: Creative nursing in day and night care centers, American Journal of Nursing 62:86-90, Sept. 1962.

Jones, Maxwell: The therapeutic community, New York, 1953, Basic Books, Inc.

Lamb, Josephine T.: Freedom for patients in mental hospitals, American Journal of Nursing 58:358-360, Mar. 1958.

McCabe, Gracia S.: Cultural influences on patient behavior, American Journal of Nursing 60:1101-1104, Aug. 1960.

Morimoto, Francoise R.: Favoritism in personnel-patient interaction, Nursing Research 3:109-112, Feb. 1955.

Morimoto, Francoise R.: The socializing role of psychiatric ward personnel, American Journal of Nursing 54:53-55, Jan. 1954.

Pearce, Helen E.: The patients tell their story, American Journal of Nursing 61:97, April 1961.

Ruhlman, Rose G. and Ishiyama, Toaru: Remedy for the forgotten back ward, American Journal of Nursing 64:109-111, July 1964.

Sabshin, Melvin: Nurse-doctor-patient relationships in psychiatry, American Journal of Nursing 57:188-192, Feb. 1957.

Sommer, Robert: Working effectively with groups, American Journal of Nursing 60:223-226, Feb. 1960.

Stanton, Alfred H.: The mental hospital, New York, 1954, Basic Books, Inc.

Stevens, Leonard F.: What makes a ward climate therapeutic? American Journal of Nursing 61:95-96, Mar. 1961.

Von Mering, Otto, and King, Stanley H.: Remotivating the mental patient, New York, 1957, Russell Sage Foundation.

Nursing care of patients with functional deviate behavior patterns

Chapter X

Nursing care of patients with withdrawal patterns

The behavior pattern characterized by withdrawal has as its central theme the refusal to invest emotional energy or attach any enduring emotional interest to persons or objects outside the self. Depending upon past experience and the incorporated standards of behavior of significant other people, withdrawal may vary widely in degree and widely in its method of expression. In other words, withdrawn behavior is not a simple, clear-cut diagnostic category. It is essential to understand that many forms of behavior exemplify the withdrawal pattern, and it is the basic failure to externalize emotional attachment that is the significant starting point of difficulties. In addition, the compensation developed to overcome the threat to security growing out of the resultant loneliness may take different forms with different individuals. The compensatory mechanisms will, however, carry through consistently the withholding of emotional investment in the environment.

The failure to respond to external situations or to invest anything in the environment leads to inconsistencies in behavior that appear as rather complete personality disorganization. Most person's behavior, viewed from the outside, holds at least some degree of reasonableness in the eye of the viewer. In the withdrawn person, thinking and emotional and action responses may differ from each other and be inappropriate to the situation. The failure to respond behaviorally to the checks and balances of reality results in actions and expressions that are difficult for the uninitiated, and many times the initiated, to understand.

Dynamics of development

The early self-organization of withdrawn individuals is self-depreciatory in nature, causing a marked feeling of insecurity in interpersonal relationships. Patients who develop this pattern tend to come from family situations characterized by conflict, tension, and anxiety. In an anxiety-laden home, the child has difficulty in building a self-image that gives him

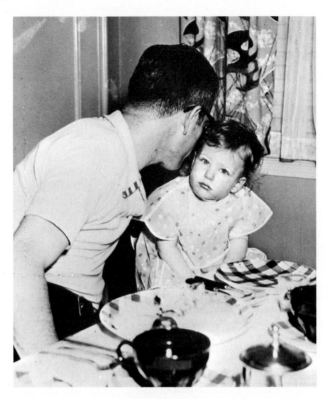

The attitudes of a child toward herself are derived from her parents' attitudes toward her.

confidence in himself as a person with an identity of his own, in developing trust in others, and in learning techniques for relating to others that contribute to his security. He sees himself as unable to function comfortably with others and sees others as a source of anxiety. Through this combination of events, security is grossly undermined and a certain compensatory indifference or independence toward the environment develops. Under such circumstances, strong motivational systems which cannot be expressed or accepted are dissociated from the self-system. The biologic and social tendencies to interact with others and expand into one's environment have no outlet for the energy associated with them, and this energy or emotional capacity must be invested in the self. This makes the achievement of maturity, in which the satisfactions and security of another can be as important as the individual's own, almost impossible. Narcissism, or self-love, becomes thoroughly embedded in the personality.

The end result is an introverted personality whose interests are directed toward the self and whose satisfactions are derived from within the self. Because of his narcissism, such a person is extremely sensitive, and the world often becomes an unpleasant place to live. Immobilization, in a sense, occurs as a protective device, and the self-organization tends to become more and more rigid. As this occurs, the person is less able to integrate the newness in any situation, and any change in the personality growth toward health is less likely to happen spontaneously.

Since the achievement of security is the immediate goal and life itself is so painful that security seems impossible, the intellect becomes a tool for rationalization and fogging of reality rather than a tool for reason and adaptation to reality. The reality principle, or testing of behavior and emotion against the actual situation with its potential consequences, fades in importance.

The conflict between success and the struggle necessary to achieve it continues, and withdrawal from reality follows withdrawal of emotional investment in the environment. Difficulties accumulate. The less realistic an individual is, the more unfortunate are his attempts to establish interpersonal relationships with others. Since personality is not static, but dynamic, its development must go in some direction. The present is a painfully insurmountable barrier to the future, and the only choice open is to retreat. Regression follows, and the individual sinks progressively lower toward earlier stages of experience and behavior patterns. The pattern of regression may affect the total personality or may affect only certain aspects of it. When this process reaches the stage that social standards have no meaning, primitive behavior makes its appearance. There is total personality disorganization, with autistic speech, confusion, and inappropriate behavior, and the dissociated self may be given independent power and even rule the self.

Particularly significant is the life history of such patients. One has not yet been found who has had a happy childhood. With a built-in lack of self-respect as a result of fairly consistent and unfortunate early experience, successive life crises are faced with increasing apprehension and increasing failures. Such persons tend to complete the break with reality in puberty or early adulthood and follow a pattern of progressive maladjustment.

The course of the development of a withdrawal type of mental illness is not so even or steadily forward as here described. This is simply an overall view. There are irregularities that occur, steps forward and backward, until some crisis precipitates a disorganization of the self. Although this may appear to be quite sudden and inexplicable to persons close to the patient, there are usually signs that indicate that trouble is developing long before the actual illness is seen. The significance of these signs is usually missed. In addition, they do not always follow a classical pattern of development that is easy to identify. Textbook pictures of clinical illness in psychiatry are the exception rather than the rule.

Range of behavior

The symptoms that are shown by a patient who becomes mentally ill are an indication of what is happening to his self-organization and its integration with others. Persons with a normal introverted personality do exist, and many get along well without serious difficulties. Intellectual achievement may bring sufficient social approval as compensation. Experience that is corrective with significant people may integrate into the introverted personality a core of warmth that may support it well. Environmental stress may not be sufficient to precipitate a breakdown. In addition, experience is not often consistent enough to produce a "pure" introvert. Most persons are a mixture of introversion and extroversion. If the introversion, however, is markedly predominant, and experience *does* produce a disorganization of the self, it will probably be in the direction of withdrawal from reality to the realm of intellectual phantasy.

The patient's pattern of behavior is usually an indication of the illness that is to follow. There will usually have been past difficulty in socialization with others, many times in combination with a quiet, studious well-behaved exterior. Such persons tend to daydream much, and, if they are outstanding in any area, it is usually in the intellectual field.

Physically such patients do not show a consistent pattern of any type of defect although some of them do not seem generally well equipped to meet life adequately on a physical basis. The implications of this fact are uncertain since what positive findings have been shown, such as irregularities in carbohydrate metabolism and poor vasomotor control, are not consistent, nor can the findings be shown positively to be either cause or effect. Considerable work has been done in the last sixty years exploring the possible underlying causes of the withdrawal pattern of behavior. Genetic inadequacy, biochemical disturbance, family influences, cultural influences, and psychologic factors have been areas of study, but none of the intensive studies has produced conclusive evidence. Current thinking leans toward psychologic causation, with early life experience, family life, and cultural factors considered especially significant. More evidence is needed than we now have before any conclusions are definite.

Recently, there was considerable hope aroused when it was thought that the administration of certain experimental drugs, such as D-lysergic acid and mescaline, produced typical responses that resembled the psychotic symptoms of the withdrawn patient. This pointed toward a biochemical causation. However, further research tied the results achieved by the administration of such medications to the familiar toxic psychoses rather than the withdrawal pattern of behavior. D-lysergic acid, an ergot derivative known as LSD, along with psilocybin, have been used experimentally in therapy although there is a strong controversy over the use of the so-called consciousness-expanding drugs.

The symptoms shown by withdrawn patients are the result of regression which results in evidences of the following: (1) autistic thinking, characteristic of infancy, when self and environment are not clearly distinguished, and meaning is highly personal in character; (2) lack of influence of reality and thus no check on behavior that would ordinarily be inhibited; and (3) inability to distinguish between a symbol and the thing

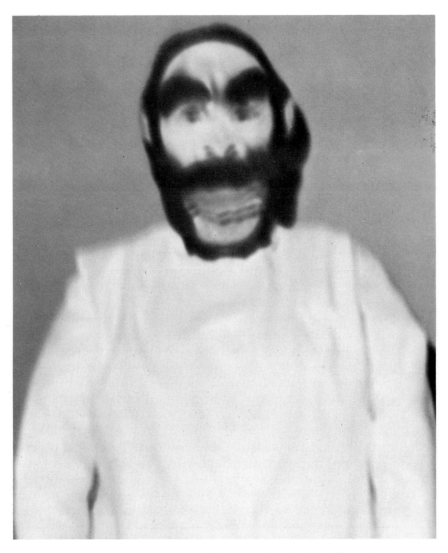

The reality perception of withdrawn patients is often distorted.

symbolized. *How* this will be expressed will depend upon the past experience of the individual. The reason we do not see the actual behavior of an infant is that the patient carries back with him in his regression the tools of adult living, such as language, which are then misused on an infantile level. In addition, certain integrated parts of the personality from higher levels may persist.

The gross interference with the function of personality is shown in motor behavior, in intellectual activity, and in emotional responses. Behavior may show a complete indifference to surroundings, and the patient will be content to sit alone and daydream. Symbolic, ritualistic dancing or posturing may express primitive or sexual wishes. Behavior may show an active resistance to any form of suggestion or influence from the environment. There may be periods of overactivity which may or may not be wholly impulsive and seem usually purposeless to the observer. Common to all of these patients is the rejection of reality and its loss of influence on conduct. Social criteria do not apply.

Emotional responses may be inadequate, inappropriate, and apathetic, or the patient may show extreme tension which is discharged in sudden bursts of overactivity. The patient may show these reactions in combination or in sequence or may show one type of reaction consistently. These emotional responses can be understood if we remember that the patient is feeling at an autistic level, where experience has its own personal meaning, unchecked by reality, and that both the self-system and the dissociated self are being expressed rather openly and often independently.

Intellectual disorders are rich in numbers and content. Events are interpreted in terms of autistic phantasy, rather than in the actual situation in which they occur. Association is, of course, disrupted. Ideas may be fused or condensed, resulting in neologisms, or the creation of new words. Consent and girl may become conirl. Ideas and language may be highly symbolic, and one word may carry the meaning of an entire experience. Skidding, or the lack of a central idea or object, in thinking and communication may occur. Specific events or ideas may be interpreted as generalizations in application. Thinking may block suddenly or may be impoverished. There may be omissions in the chain of sequence of thought. This may go so far as complete incoherence or lack of any integration in the intellectual processes. In addition, there may occur certain disorders of content of thought, the most important of these symptoms being delusions and hallucinations. Delusions are fixed false beliefs, out of keeping with one's background, beliefs which cannot be altered by reason or experience. This can happen as a result of the patient's escape from the principle of reality as a guide for behavior. Hallucinations are imaginary sense perceptions and can occur in any of the five senses, although auditory and visual hallucinations are the most common. It must be remembered that the patient has regressed to an autistic stage, in which the differentiation between self and notself is no longer clear. In addition, projection operates here, as well as the fact that the self and the dissociated self are independent personalities.

No patient shows all of these disorders but weaves varying patterns both as to objective manifestations of behavior and content of subjective experience.

There may be or may not be an active stage of the illness in which the patient shows marked emotional stress and active efforts to reintegrate himself into his environment, bizarrely unfortunate though such behavior may be. It is however, a good sign since this conflict period may be resolved by a return to mental health. The patient at least is not indifferent or apathetic toward his environment. Such an active withdrawal holds promise for recovery. The patient who withdraws passively, showing increasing apathy and flatness or blunting of the emotional response, is a more difficult therapuetic problem.

Some patients simply show a lack of interest, are totally devoid of ambition, and drift whither circumstances send them. They respond but little to social criteria, and their emotional lives are superficial since they form no real or enduring attachments to anything or anyone. Their passive course does not carry through to bizarre enough behavior to attract undue attention. The village ne'er-do-wells, the town drunkards, hobos, prostitutes, and the bowery bums number many such persons among their camaraderie. A general belief is held that this group does not respond well to treatment, but it is difficult to so state categorically since only a small percent of them ever come under treatment.

There may occur a sudden, violent upheaval characterized by silliness, grimacing, posturing, delusions, and hallucinations of fantastic or grotesque nature. Behavior may be markedly impulsive and emotional response totally inappropriate. The strong emotional response usually dies out fairly quickly.

Another form occurs in which conduct peculiarity is marked. The patient swings from periods of stupor to excitement. There occur impulsive but stereotyped behavior, hallucinations, and a strong negativistic reaction to all suggestion from the environment. The patient approaches the area of magic here, and identifies with cosmic forces. They are the battleground of good and evil. During periods of stupor, the patient maintains a rigidly assumed position and shows the famous waxy flexibility that is *almost* diagnostic. He will hold rigidly, and for hours on end, a position in which he is placed. The excited period tends to be explosive, and sudden attacks on the environment or self are fairly common.

A coloring of projection may be added to the form of illness in that any of these patients may develop suspiciousness and fear of the intent of the environment. Traits from one of the three types briefly described may appear in either of the other two types, but a particular behavior pattern will usually predominate.

Nursing care

The bizarre and seemingly illogical behavior of patients who have rejected reality seems often so incomprehensible to the average nurse that she is bewildered as to what her function in the care of such patients may be. Analysis of the patient's behavior will indicate certain needs that are paramount in combating his illness. The focus must be placed on the patient as a person, rather than on the symptoms he shows. Actually one of the most challenging nursing problems that exists is to help back to healthy social participation the patient who has emphatically turned his back on interpersonal relationships and the society in which he lives. It is not easy.

Psychotherapeutic environment. The recovery of a patient with a severe withdrawal pattern of behavior must be based on reeducation of his perception of himself in relation to others. First, he must be able to see himself as he is, lose his negative attitude toward himself, and rebuild a new perception in its place. Normal society has failed to accomplish this; therefore a new type of existence, oriented to make possible such reeducation, is indicated.

Security is one of the patient's first and greatest needs so that his opinion of himself is supported consistently, and no demand that he cannot meet is presented to him. The physical environment can contribute in several ways. A limited physical range provides the security of sameness upon which the patient can depend. A routine that is reasonably the same day by day contributes to security, as does the limited number of persons the patient comes in contact with in the hospital. In order to be effective, a routine should provide sameness; yet it should have enough variety not to be monotonous. This is particularly important since the patient's tendency to withdraw and to regress can be supported by institutional routines. Every effort should be made to keep the patient focused in the direction of everyday life.

The routine should also include some activities that do not lend themselves readily to stereotyped performances and that cannot be carried through without attention or thought. Attention to reality is important. The physical set-up should be clean and cheerful to provide stimulation on a pleasant level of reality. If the patient's withdrawal is an active form of rejection, the environment should be restricted to permit tactful observation and to limit the possibilities of destructiveness toward others or self.

In a psychologic sense the hospital environment offers the patient several advantages. He is removed from significant persons around whom his difficulties may center. He is relieved of the necessity for making decisions and of the many demands of day-by-day existence. He can be comfortably ill because in the new setting that is what is expected of him and because his behavior is not particularly unusual in the new culture. He is accepted as he is. Failure does not face him at every turn; judgment is not pronounced against him.

Interpersonal relationships. Fundamentally, the most important part of a patient's environment is the people around him. Good psychiatric nursing can be practiced almost anywhere. In the hospital setting, the persons in authority are quite significant, including the nurses who determine when one will arise and go to bed, when one will eat, and where one will go and why. For the most part the nurses and the persons who work on the floor with patients determine the psychologic atmosphere in which the patient will live. They support or undermine the therapeutic program.

Certain problems in the establishment of interpersonal relationships with such patients are characteristic of withdrawal patterns of behavior.

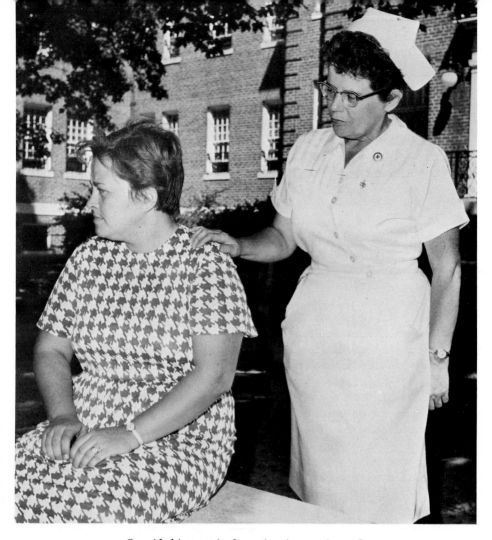

One-sided interest in the patient is a nursing tool.

Healthy, interpersonal relationships cannot of course be established at once, and, in fact, any establishment is the immediate problem. However, from the beginning an attempt can be made to build rapport on a foundation that will lend itself to healthy growth by the patient.

The first and most important problem is to reach the patient emotionally and establish some bond. In view of the patient's rejection of people, it can readily be seen that the initiative must rest with personnel. It must be a consistent, steady attempt to draw the patient into some response, without, at the same time, demanding any response. The patient *must* be left free to respond because he wishes to. This means one-sided conversations, one-sided interest in the patient's appearance, and one-sided interest in everything the patient does. Such a program must be carried through for a long period, always sincerely and always without any retaliation by word, posture, gesture, or attitude for the patient's failure to respond. When a response does come, mature techniques of social skill should not be expected, and the patient's fumbling and often inept social responses should be accepted with the same grace and tolerance with which indifference was accepted. At the same time, the response must be recognized for what it is, a step in the right direction. Sudden verbal lashings, incoherent language, grimacing, and absurd and silly behavior would be expected. It is wise to remember that the labels given such behavior in the immediately preceding sentence reflect our judgments which must not be referred to the patient. Could we understand the meaning of his behavior as it appears to him, the patient might well be justified in reversing the judgment and applying it to us.

The problem of verbal communication is no easy one. The patient uses language in a highly personal way and has his own individual meaning for words, phrases, and sentences. Experience unchecked by reality may be quite distorted, and fantasy may reign unchecked. Therefore, if the patient shows such symptoms, it is wise to keep communication directed toward him in simple language. Also, it must be remembered that communication occurs on more than verbal and intellectual levels and that emotional communication may be even more important in this instance. The constant awareness and seeking out of the patient at every opportunity communicates the nurse's interest. Sitting quietly beside a patient saying nothing for brief but consistent periods conveys its message. It is wise not to get trapped in the patient's intellectual fantasies, not to argue about them, and not to attempt to reason them away. Acceptance of the patient without criticism and without ignoring him does not necessarily sanction his behavior. However, the withdrawn person must be sought— he will not seek others.

Certain types of behavior shown by such patients have a tendency to try the nurse's control because of cultural attitudes of disgust that are deeply ingrained in most of us. Since reality has little meaning, social standards have none for such patients. Careless personal exposure, indiscriminate defecation, and carelessness in regard to personal appearance and odors tend to arouse strong disapproval. Such behavior should be seen as a mark of regression and an indication of the degree of the patient's illness. Such behavior would be in keeping with that of a very small child— and the withdrawn patient may well regress to that level. Quiet acceptance without prudishness or open expression of disgust is indicated. Experience helps.

In all relationships with such patients, the core of all efforts must be centered around the attempt to build the patient's badly shattered opinion of himself. Encouragement and praise may be used, but only when they are justified and can be accepted by the patient. After all, the most important thing another person can do for us is to be interested in us. That in itself, if it is consistent, helps. Although praise and encouragement may be used, their reverse, criticism and admonishment, should never be. The sensitive ego must be nourished carefully. Until it has been rebuilt, it cannot tolerate the little rebuffs and the give-and-take of ordinary relationships.

Physical needs. In line with the patient's isolation and indifference to the usual social criteria, certain physical problems follow. The responsibility for personal cleanliness and personal appearance falls on the nurse. Attention to such particulars should be cared for without making the patient conspicuous because it must be done for him. Attention to personal appearance may result in some expression of approval from group members, which is good for the patient.

Since the physical capacities of many such patients are not great, careful attention to nutrition, elimination, and adequate exercise are indicated. Close observation for any signs of physical illness is necessary since many patients will not report their physical difficulties. Prompt and careful attention to physical illnesses is important.

Protection. Certain protective needs of patients with withdrawal patterns grow out of their particular symptom syndrome. Since their intellectual processes tend to digress from routine and expected patterns, the degree of predictability in regard to their behavior is reduced. Hence behavior that seems purposeless and impulsive to the outside observer can and frequently does occur. Patients need alert and imaginative observation to protect them from the possible consequences of impulsive and unself-disciplined acts. Sudden attacks on others, often without any evident personal animosity, can occur, as well as sudden jumps or wall-diving that may result in personal injury or death.

Patients need also to be protected from possible group consequences as a result of their indifference to social standards exhibited through exposure, profanity, or crude sexual gestures. During periods when behavior along such lines is prevalent, it may be necessary to temporarily isolate the patient from the group. Withdrawn patients also need protection, both physically and psychologically, from others in the environment who are more aggressive. As a rule it is much wiser to anticipate such a need and move to meet it before any incident actually occurs.

One of the patient's great needs is to be protected from idleness and unbridled indulgence in phantasy. An effort to keep the patient actively participating in life within the hospital routine and at some task that requires a contact with reality must always be made.

Group relations. Withdrawn patients pose some real problems in relationships with other members of the group in the hospital unit. A predominance of passively withdrawn patients can hold a group interaction to a depressive minimum, and a predominance of actively withdrawn patients can completely disrupt a group. As a minority within a group, they tend individually to be isolates. Although they perhaps are not verbally interacting with other patients, nonetheless they are definitely part of the group emotionally, and their presence has its effect on other members, and other members affect the withdrawn patient. Participation occurs on other levels than verbal.

In group relations, the withdrawn patient is always in danger of attack from more aggressive patients. The latter may need a safe outlet for their aggression and realize the withdrawn patient presents it, or they may feel a resentment of the withdrawn patient's seeming lack of pressure of activity which plagues the aggressive patient himself. If the group comes to the patient's defense, well and good; the action then conveys an acceptance of the patient which he needs whether he can acknowledge it or not. In such an instance, the aggressive patient needs help. If, however, it falls upon the nurse to rescue the withdrawn patient, she must do so tactfully through diversion of the aggressive patient. To openly champion the quieter person may isolate him further from the group.

When a patient is being guided to participate in socialized activities, encouragement and support are useful. The patient may be placed with another patient, much like himself to start with, and then the two are later fitted into a slightly larger group containing perhaps more active members. The members of the group should remain fairly constant if possible, unless the group reaction is unfortunate. In regard to activity within the group, the particular form of occupation chosen for or by the patient may be something he can do alone. Shared activities may be introduced later, with the element of competition held to a minimum, until the patient seems comfortable in the group.

The nurse should at all times avoid placing her relationship with the patient on a footing that isolates him from the group of patients. Competition for her favors will occur, and behavior that results in rejection of the patient by others deprives him of one of the real values of hospitalization.

Convalescence. During the convalescent period, the withdrawn person usually needs further support for his ego and reassurance in regard to his return to society. One of the best ways to develop an objective attitude toward his mental illness is through the nurse's own matter-of-fact, objective acceptance of it. The patient should be allowed to talk through his feelings about going home if he wishes without having them treated lightly. Socialized activities should be encouraged, and the patient should be given opportunities to develop social skills until he feels relatively sure of himself if possible. Bridge, dancing, and other activities that can be enjoyably shared should be practiced until they can be done well, on the simple principle that most persons enjoy doing what they can do well, and the withdrawn patient's greatest need is for things he can do well with others.

Attention should be focused on the value of day-by-day experience and the acquirement of good health habits, including a balanced program of work and play. Realistic ideas concerning future plans should be supported; unrealistic ideas should not be criticized but left to the patient to talk through and evaluate. Requested information should be given freely on the level of the patient's understanding, and advice should be abjured.

The patient should be given gradual and increased responsibility for himself and his decisions so that he begins to outgrow his dependence before he leaves the hospital. In addition, this is an excellent period for learning from the patient, for most patients have some skill, knowledge, or understanding which they can impart. Let them give.

References

Andrews, Dixie: A process recording on a schizophrenic-hebephrenic patient, Perspectives in psychiatric care 1:11-39, Nov. 1963.

Arieti, Silvana: Schizophrenia. In Arieti, Silvana, editor: Handbook of american psychiatry, New York, 1959, Basic Books, Inc., vol. 1, pp. 455-507.

Carl, Mary Kathryn: Establishing a relationship with a schizophrenic patient, Perspectives in Psychiatric Care 1:20-22, Mar.-Apr. 1963.

Ewalt, Jack R. and Farnsworth, Dana L.: Textbook of psychiatry, New York, 1963, McGraw-Hill Book Co., Inc., pp. 207-231.

Field, William E.: When a patient hallucinates, American Journal of Nursing 63:80-82, Feb. 1963.

Goodman, Lillian R.: Regression, Nursing Outlook 10:265-267, April 1962.

Goodman, Lillian R. and LaBelle, Mary J.: The schizophrenic's mother, Nursing Outlook 11:753-754, Oct. 1963.

Hurtcau, Phyllis, The psychiatric nurse and the mute patient, American Journal of Nursing 62:55-60, June 1962.

Jackson, Don D.: Schizophrenia, Scientific American 207:65-74, Aug. 1962.

Noyes, Arthur P. and Kolb, Lawrence C.: Modern Clinical Psychiatry, ed. 6, Philadelphia, 1963, W. B. Saunders Co., pp. 325-364.

Robinson, Alice M.: Communication with schizophrenic patients, American Journal of Nursing 60:1120-1123, Aug. 1960.

Schwartz, Charlotte Green, Schwartz, Morris S., and Stanton, Alfred H.: A study of need-fulfillment on a mental hospital ward, Psychiatry 14:223-242, May 1951.

Schwartz, Morris S., and Shockley, Emmy Lanning: The nurse and the mental patient, New York, 1956, Russell Sage Foundation, pp. 90-138.

Schwartz, Morris S., and Will, Gwen Tudor: Low morale and mutual withdrawal on a mental hospital ward, Psychiatry 16:337-353, Nov. 1953.

Sullivan, Harry Stack: Conceptions of modern psychiatry, Washington, D. C., 1947, William Alanson White Psychiatric Foundation, pp. 71-84.

Tudor, Gwen: A sociopsychiatric nursing approach to intervention in a problem of mutual withdrawal on a mental hospital ward, Psychiatry 15:193-217, May 1952.

Van Huben, Betty J.: Discussion of a process recording on a schizophrenic-hebephrenic patient, Perspectives in Psychiatric Care 1:40-44, Nov. 1963.

Chapter xi

Nursing care of patients with aggressive patterns

There exists a group of reaction patterns in which overt behavior is characterized by reactions which seemingly are markedly different but which experience and study have shown to be closely related. This constellation is characterized by disturbances in affect, usually exaggerations in varying degrees of normal moods. The behavior organization, although obviously deviating from accepted social standards, remains on a higher level than is seen in the personality disruption that accompanies withdrawal. The basic personalities possess much in common, the areas of vulnerability are similar, and, in some cases, the varying methods of seeking resolutions may be substituted for each other or follow each other in a definite sequence. The related patterns include behavior showing explosive excitement, behavior showing retarded depression, and behavior showing agitated depression with some of the characteristics of the other two.

Dynamics of development

Early childhood experience and acquired self-organization and direction of personality growth are important. A potential patient does not experience the devastating childhood that marks the history of a withdrawn patient. He does, however, undergo experiences which force upon him the necessity for continuously struggling to achieve security and a sense of confidence in his own self-esteem through relationships with others. He early loses a loved one either in reality or symbolically, usually by the withdrawal of close or intense care that had been given him previously. At the time of the withdrawal or reduction of care, increased demands were made upon him. This produced compliance and a struggle for approval on his part, along with resentment against the demands and the resultant self-negation. In response to the aroused resentment and the fear of failure to achieve desired acceptance, feelings of guilt are aroused. The sequence of events becomes hostility and a sense of guilt. Since the self-system tends to integrate those elements of any experience or situation to which the person has become sensitized, future experiences that produce considerable tension and growing self-doubt may be considered the vulnerable point of such a personality. Situations that are particularly significant for such individuals are the loss of a valued object, for example, a loved one or a job, or the realization of an empty kind of existence.

Although the central problem of such persons is handling the hostility and the accompanying feelings of guilt that result from threats to security, it must be noted that the total response or absolute direction of the personality is not hostilely oriented. There are more positive emotional responses available that result in ambivalence, or existence of two opposite emotions at the same time. The person both loves and hates a significant other person for whom he has affection or respect. The same may occur in regard to a significant part of experience, such as the ability to hold a job which has an important meaning for the individual. The job may produce some forms of experience which threaten security and self-esteem and call forth an ambivalent emotional response.

It may well be that the incorporation of a positive personality aspect within such a person enables him to maintain a better personality organization and more nearly normal behavior patterns when and if he is overwhelmed by life situations. This may be an important reason for the difference between the prognosis for a withdrawal pattern of behavior and an aggressive pattern of behavior.

When a personality with such a vulnerable aspect is exposed to prolonged tension or anxiety involving a strong threat to his self-esteem or a significant loss, he may respond in one of several ways. Having been so schooled, his hostility, a natural response to a threat, calls forth feelings of guilt, and he resorts to the mechanism of dealing with hostility that was inculcated in him by early experience. His conscience, his superego, or his introjected parental role, as you may wish to name it, is called into action. He may not resist the savage derogation it inflicts, but seek to reinforce it. In such instances, he will feel an overwhelming anxiety that is expressed in self-delusions of unpardonable sinfulness that threaten the self and may threaten everyone and that grows into an impending sense of world disaster. This core of ideas becomes a preoccupation. Such reinforcement of the self-condemnatory attitude results in agitated depression.

The individual may accept the derogatory self-estimate passively, and the delusional reaction may then be centered on his self-inadequacies and failures, rather than on his crimes. Guilt and unworthiness are accepted, and the individual is hopeless and helpless. Such an attitude tends to result in retarded depression. Feelings of sadness, unworthiness, and hopelessness are accompanied by physical slowness and retardation. Both agitated and retarded depressions are methods of self-punishment—hostility finds its outlet on the self.

The other reaction to the derogatory self-evaluation is an aggressive one, which usually overcompensates by open rebellion against the edict. Aggressive self-assertion is shown by an attempt to dominate the environment through sheer activity. The underlying tension and hostility are expressed in frantic activity, in outbursts of destructiveness, in the use of ridicule, and in rage at any restriction or obstacle.

The root of these disorders is in the personality, which has strong ambivalent tendencies toward introjection and susceptibility toward dependency on significant persons in the environment, a sensitivity to self-doubt, and a fear of the expression of hostility which any threat to security arouses. A patient may show a mixture of patterns, may follow one type of reaction with another, or may show only one type of reaction. The basic reaction is an aggressive one and may be either directed on the environment or turned inward upon the self.

There has been a great deal of conjecture concerning the relationship of this type of disorder to somatic build, heredity, and biochemical function. Some investigations have also been made into related social and cultural factors. Although none of the work has been conclusive beyond question, two fairly well accepted ideas in general practice have been the following: (1) heredity does play some part in the incidence of affective psychoses although what part is not clear, and (2) social and cultural factors do play a part in the development of such disorders. It is also generally accepted that the occurrence of a depression is related to a significant loss, real or symbolic, on the part of the patient. It is interesting to note that affective disorders are decreasing as cultural changes take place in the United States. It is also interesting to note that this type of disorder tends to occur more frequently in the upper social classes than in the lower social classes. What this means is fuel for speculation at the present.

Range of behavior

The types of behavior shown by persons with these personality disorders is perhaps a little easier to understand than some forms of mental illness. The patterns of underactivity and overactivity are ones into which normal persons can project themselves with a little imagination. In addition such patients are much easier to communicate with, and one can follow their verbal expression. Less exaggerated forms of agitation, retardation, and excitement are common experiences to all people. Everyone worries and feels tension and anxiety, which tends to spread from one situation to another. Anxiety regarding one's competence in business may spread to anxiety concerning one's home. New doubts are added, and one may feel depressed, sad, and lonely. Activity and initiative slow up; mild agitation may result, or active and enforced gaiety may be used to cover up or dispel the feelings. Such responses in exaggeration become personality disorders.

Any of the deviations are usually precipitated by situations threatening enough to security to produce anxiety and tension over a long period. As indicated before, this is often related to the loss of a valued object, which can have varied meanings, including another person, a significant possession, a job, or one's own sense of competence.

A frequent precipitating factor in agitated depressions, for example, is the climacteric which marks the beginning of the process of aging. The loss of sexual and socioeconomic status is a threat to self-esteem.

The agitated depression is exactly what it says—a depressed emotional state accompanied by increased motor activity. Restlessness is characteristic, and activity is continual but limited in range. The patient paces back and forth wringing her hands, picking at her skin, and biting her nails. She is overwhelmed by a group of ideas or delusions of worthlessness, poverty, unreality, and sinfulness. She is completely preoccupied with this core of ideas centered about her sense of self-depreciation and self-reproach. She dreads the deserved punishment that awaits her and bitterly regrets the impending disaster she has brought on others. In the course of her illness she has neither the time nor the effort for sleep and food. Indecisiveness and uncooperativeness are common. The need for punishment is so deep that the danger of suicide is very real.

The retarded depression is again exactly what it says—a depressed emotional state accompanied by a slowing down or retarding of thinking processes and motor activity. There is first a general slowing up that is accompanied by a feeling of sadness and dejection and a loss of initiative. Anxiety and tension persist throughout the episode although their presence may be masked by later symptoms. A loss of weight occurs, and physical movements become slow and require much effort. The stream of thought becomes restricted and centers on ideas and delusions of personal unworthiness, self-depreciation, and convictions of failure in the past and the future. Thinking requires much effort, and only a limited range of ideas and simple thoughts can be handled. There is difficulty in concentrating on anything other than the hopeless and helpless ideas of self-rejection. Sitting in idleness, the head bowed and the face worn and haggard, the patient painfully endures his self-depreciation. He sleeps little and eats poorly. Practically the entire metabolic process is slowed down. The danger of suicide in this instance is greatest as the patient goes into and comes out of his depression.

The excitement pattern is shown by elation or aggressive self-assertion which may reach delusional proportions. Delusions are usually fleeting and expansive, even grandiose, in nature. An energetic overactivity is displayed in which the patient rushes into reality and keeps himself preoccupied with his environment. The attention span is limited, and there is little ability to follow through or carry to completion any activity or thought. Focus of attention shifts so rapidly that a flight of ideas of varying degrees may occur. The patient may reach a goal idea by a devious roundabout pathway or may never reach it at all.

The flight of ideas may be shown by a quick reference to the objects or persons the patients sees or by quick jumps in ideas associated with the words used. Rhyming, punning, quips, and various witticisms may be seen. A general tendency to express openly primitive or purely biologic impulses is evidenced, and vulgarity and obscenity are common. The overac-

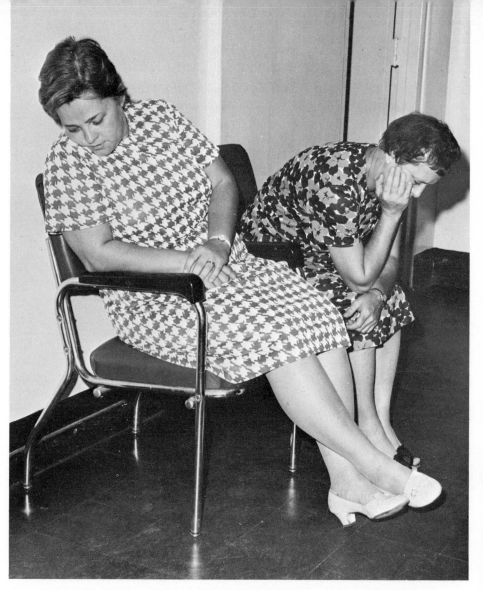

Mental depression is reflected in physical appearance and reduced motor activity.

tivity may include singing, shouting, and dancing. The patient often teases others and acts the clown. Through all this performance runs an impulsiveness that may include destructiveness such as attacks on others. Irritability is usually marked, and the patient tolerates restrictions and restraints very poorly. Food, rest, and elimination are neglected, and the patient becomes dehydrated and loses weight. He is a ready prey to infections of any kind.

These three related syndromes are the most important of the aggressive reaction patterns. As has been pointed out, any combination of these patterns may occur, and they may include behavior not here described. There is a common tendency among these patients for both self-limiting episodic attacks and recurring attacks. The recovery rate from individual attacks is very high, but the high rate of recurrence reduces the hopeful outlook for the future to some extent.

Nursing care

The nursing care of the patient with aggressive behavior, directed outwardly as well as inwardly, differs somewhat in the specific types of nursing problems likely to be presented. The pattern of illness, with its typical acute episodes that tend to be self-limited and also recurrent, suggests a plan for treatment that fits the episodic nature. Psychotherapy under the physician's direction takes advantage of the patient's better periods and concentrates on constructive interrelationships during the acute period to establish a good foundation for the later and more intensive psychic probing that will take place. The procedure is significant in its implications for nursing care.

Psychotherapeutic environment. The essence of a psychotherapeutic environment for overactive and depressed patients is that it be unchallenging and nonstimulating. A quietly pleasant ward, in physical appearance and in psychologic atmosphere, is necessary. Noise should be kept to a minimum, irritation avoided at all costs, and the administration of ward routine guided by the patient's needs. The restrictive elements of routine, if they exist, such as counting patients and locking doors, should be eliminated or should be done as tactfully and quickly as possible. Allowance should be made for the slowness of depressed patients and the impulsive, distractable inefficiency of overactive patients. Since the underlying problem of hostility must be considered, the environment should restrict as far as possible the opportunities for its expression to be disastrous. The fact that stimulation can result from such varied things as bright colors, tension in others, a routine too closely calculated in regard to time, fatigue, noise, lack of outlet for energy, and numerous other factors should be taken into account when patient care is planned, both administratively and individually.

Facilities for the treatment of symptoms that are uncomfortable for the patient should be readily available. Overactivity feeds on overactivity and can set in motion a vicious cycle which leaves a patient exhausted and overstimulated by his own fatigue.

The advent of tranquilizers has reduced markedly the extent to which actual patient control is a problem.

Interpersonal relationships. Aggressive patients need contact with persons who can accept them as they are and who function as rather neutral but human buffers who accept them and against whom they can test themselves without retaliation or judgment. Patients must be able to express their hostility and ambivalence in a calm accepting atmosphere in which their guilt is not reinforced. The limitations placed on them by their symptoms must not be used against them.

The overactive patient presents certain problems in interpersonal relationships. He is too active physically and has, therefore, a high nuisance value; he resents authority; he tends to be domineering; he is sarcastic and fond of ridicule; he enjoys embarrassing others; he is impulsive; he has a limited attention span; his sense of humor is often crude; his wit and verbal punning is often too funny; he demands attention and will not be ignored; he is profane and vulgar; and he is very sensitive. What does such a person need in his relationship with others?

Above all, he needs a person with good self-control who can see and understand objectively what is happening to him. He needs a person who can be calm and collected under all or most circumstances and whose judgment can surmount the annoyances of the patient's behavior. The answer lies in the ability to accept a person without necessarily sanctioning his behavior. This can be done in the following manner. The patient should first of all be protected from overstimulation. His resentment of the necessary restrictions of a psychiatric hospital should be respected by limiting him tactfully and by allowing him to verbalize his annoyance. Critical comments should be matter-of-factly met, and no attempt should be made to "talk him out of it"; his verbal attacks on personnel should not be met with self-defense or explanation. One of the favorite traps in an overactive patient's attack on his environment is to force personnel into a defense of themselves or their behavior or weaknesses. Such attacks must again be met with a matter-of-fact tolerance, even when they sting, as they so often do. Careful fairness in treatment and attitude toward the patient must be maintained. Profanity and vulgarity should also be faced without prudishness. In summary, the aggressiveness, the resentment of authority, the criticalness, the vulgarity, and the attempt to belittle and challenge personnel are best met by a calm, matter-of-fact manner, and further hurt to the patient should be avoided by not increasing his feeling of guilt in relation to any such manifestations of behavior.

The achievement of such Olympian serenity is not an easy task and comes as a rule as the result of deliberate cultivation. A sudden verbal thrust at a weakness is not a pleasant experience, and, since she is a human being, the necessity for self-defense and retaliation is part and parcel of the nurse's personality, as well as of the patient. The criterion to apply to each situation is the question, What have I done for the patient? It may lead to control if the nurse is emotionally mature enough to apply it objectively. Another suggested criterion to apply to situations is the question, Have I required the patient to show greater emotional control than I have been able to show myself?

The problem of communication with overactive patients should take into consideration the patient's poor attention span, his distractibility, his tendency to be funny, his need to express hostility, and his sensitivity. Complicated ideas and long, involved explanations and discussions are contraindicated. Short, simple answers and comments, direct and to the point, are more effective. Rhetoric questions are often used by such patients, and silence is then best employed since the patient usually neither wants nor expects an answer and is annoyed with it. Direct commands are not well accepted, particularly if given in a sharp tone. The patient is easily distracted, and this symptom should be exploited to avoid difficult situations whenever possible. In this connection, it is well to remember studies have shown that patients have a tendency to be somewhat more tolerant of psychotic behavior than personnel, and what may appear to be a difficult situation for a nurse may not seem so to other patients. This is especially true of conversations and behavior related to crudeness. When the patient's conversation is very witty or funny, it is wise to guard carefully against the tendency to encourage the patient and overstimulate him. In addition, learn carefully the distinction between laughing at and laughing with patients. Patients are acutely aware of the difference and sensitive to its implications. Fairly free verbalization of hostility as shown by sarcasm and ridicule should be tolerated by personnel since the patient needs an opportunity to share his negative emotional feelings in order to learn to evaluate them. Care should be taken in comments that rejection is not implied. Comparison of the patient with other patients or comparison of his behavior with previous days should be avoided. The statement, "I like you because you are better behaved today," is a subtle threat to withdraw approval if the patient does not continue the better behavior. Encouragement and praise should be given with tact and an awareness of the possible implications of what is said. Verbal punishment and threats are taboo. Finally, overactive patients present so many problems and so often that the temptation to an impatient response is great. Such temptation should be resisted.

As can be recognized from the description of such patients, there are limitations that must be placed on interpersonal relationships and physical activities. Limitations are necessary, but the manner of their enforcement may present difficulties. No one person, patient, nurse, or other, is ever allowed free and complete expression of his immediate wishes and wants. Limitations in a psychiatric hospital, however, are or should be determined by the patient's needs. For this type of behavior, limitations are imposed because of several important considerations. The patient should not be allowed to injure himself or others so that limitations in his behavior are determined by this criterion. An expression of his hostility and ambivalent feelings is necessary so that he is allowed to go as far in this conduct as is safe for himself and the people around him. Exhaustion is an experience he should be spared; therefore, limitations are placed on how overactive he may be in terms of this factor. Limitations should be agreed on and *consistently* enforced so that the patient has the security derived from knowing what to expect. Verbal explanations in regard to limitations are of not too much value beyond a very brief explanation. Patients will learn best by experience.

The interpersonal relationship needs of a retarded personality are again related to the patient's hostility and the guilt it has aroused within him. The perception of himself as worthless and hopeless because of his hostility, his fear of expressing it, and punishment of himself for feeling

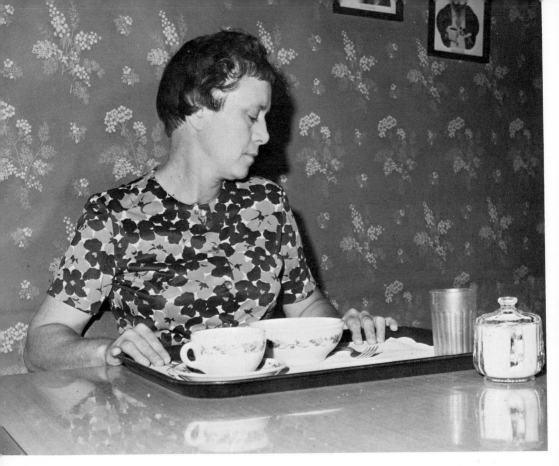

Depression is often indicated by refusal to eat.

it make the patient's nursing problems somewhat different in regard to overt behavior.

The goal in interpersonal relationship with this type of patient is to reassure the patient as to his worth as a person by making the acceptance of hostility easier for him and by reducing his deep-seated feelings of guilt. The reassurance of the patient as to his worth as a person has dual implications. First, anything that may imply by word or behavior that the patient's opinion of himself is correct should be avoided. Second, positive action can be taken that helps to build the patient's self-esteem.

Since people tend to integrate and pay attenion to the elements of experience that are pertinent to their own self-perception, the avoidance of any appearance of rejection calls for careful analysis of the behavior and attitudes of personnel. Certain characteristic situations hold specific dangers.

Life should be kept on a very simple level so that the patient is not confronted with demands he cannot meet, with resultant self-depreciation. The day's routine should be kept limited, and complex activities should be avoided. When the patient cannot care for himself, as in dressing or feeding, all necessary procedures should be done by personnel and done very matter-of-factly without reminding the patient or others that it is necessary to do things for him. Routines should allow for the patient's slowness and protect him at the same time from any attention being called to that slowness. In other words, all routine and procedures should be reduced to the limits of the patient's level of thinking and behavior without in any way making his behavior conspicuous.

Hostility and self-depreciation may be expressed either openly or symbolically and may be quietly accepted. Failure to cooperate or making extra work for personnel may indicate hostility. The rejection or active avoidance of personnel may also express it. The right to feel this way belongs to the patient, and any criticism or rejection will increase his feeling of guilt, which is already one of his central problems. His behavior, therefore, should be analyzed for elements that might be an expression of hostility, and those specific forms of behavior should be accepted calmly with special care. The patient may also seek menial tasks as an expression of his need for self-punishment and should be permitted such tasks without comment.

The patient may verbalize his feelings of worthlessness and guilt, and care should be exercised in responding to such statements. Above all, they must not be treated lightly or thrust aside as temporary manifestations which are "foolish or will disappear soon and be forgotten." They are profoundly important feelings to the patient and should be so accepted. If she is certain that the feelings rather than the intellectual content is identified, the nurse may reflect the feeling, being careful to reflect no more than the patient has expressed. For example, if the patient comments, "My mother hated me, and she had reason to because I'm no good," the patient has expressed one feeling and hinted at another, of which he is probably unaware. He feels self-depreciatory, and he is probably, judging from his expression, attributing to his mother some of his own self-judgment. Hate from his mother, real or imagined, has some emotional response and may be quite significant in the patient's illness. However, the *feeling* expressed is self-depreciation, and it is very real and important to the patient. To tell him that he is worth something is to reject him as he is, denying the importance of his feeling or implying that he should feel something else. To respond by saying, "You've felt disliked, haven't you?" accepts him, what he has said, and the feeling he has expressed. It neither condones or approves—it simply accepts. When in doubt, say nothing.

Another approach that holds depressing possibilities is an emphasis upon anything cheerful in the environment as a mistaken attempt to cheer the patient. By contrast, with such cheerfulness the patient is apt to feel more deeply depressed. The contrast of opposites in this instance is likely to be detrimental.

In addition to not adding to the patient's feelings of self-depreciation, the nurse can take steps to help the patient support a positive feeling about himself. Of course, respect for the limitations his symptoms place on him as outlined in previous paragraphs has a positive aspect. It gives evidence that the patient is respected as the person he is here and now, which is probably the most effective reassurance that can be given under any circumstances. While avoiding too much verbalization about the matter, a nurse can imply by her behavior that she feels that the patient will get well. This can be done by quiet, personalized attention to the patient, by seeking him out when routine does not demand it, and by paying attention to expressed likes and dislikes whenever possible. She can also help by not expecting the patient to appreciate what she does.

Most depressed patients have a period during the day, usually in the early evening, when their depression lifts slightly. This period of improvement should be exploited daily to reach the patient with personal interest, but should not be referred to again the next morning when the patient is more deeply depressed. Simple activities may be shared at such periods, and every effort should be made to have them as enjoyable as possible.

The goal in interpersonal relationships with patients who are agitated and depressed is approximately the same as for overactive or retarded depressed patients. However, the problems encountered in reaching the goal combine some of the elements of both types. The problems arise because of overactivity and restlessness, preoccupation with ideas of sinfulness and guilt that produce the agitation, and insistence on reassurance that cannot be accepted more than momentarily. Such a combination results in a patient to whom cooperation and diversion are almost impossible during an acute phase. Acceptance may be given as indicated previously, and care should be taken to avoid by word, attitude, or implication any rejection or depreciation of the patient, and every opportunity should be used to build the patient's self-esteem.

The agitated patient, like the overactive patient, needs a rather neutral atmosphere as a buffer although it must also be one that holds warmth and personal interest. Handling the demanded reassurances requires considerable patience and the ability to avoid impatient retorts under pressure. Impatient responses are apt to contribute to the patient's feelings of guilt.

The problem of communication centers about the patient's repeated convictions of poverty, sinfulness, etc., which usually center around a specific group of ideas. The nurse should avoid being caught in this conversational trap and keep her reassurance general rather than specific. No attempt should be made to reason the patient out of ideas that he is worse or more sinful than anyone else ever was.

It is important to reach decisions quickly and firmly for agitated patients since letting decisions hang fire by giving the patient an opportunity to make them tends to increase anxiety and tension. What is to be done must be indicated firmly and carried through at once. Explanations given must be short and specific. That diversion is not as effective as with overactive patients is indicated by resistiveness to routine and procedures

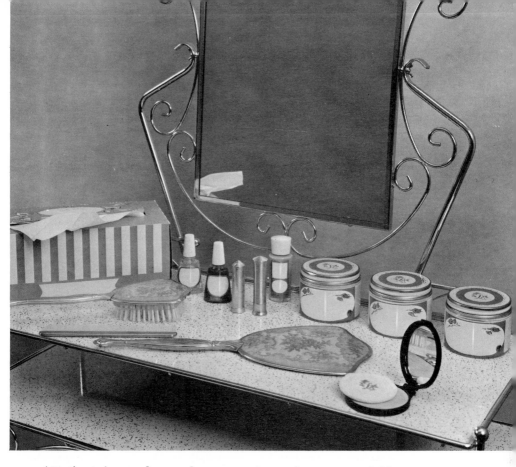

Attention to improved personal appearance is sometimes accompanied by improved mood.

which occurs because the patient is unable to attend to anything except his psychotic ideas. However, diversion should be tried.

Attention to personal appearance is often more effective with patients who show agitated depression than with patients who show retarded depression or a pattern of overactivity and therefore is an avenue of approach to be thoroughly exploited. It is also a means of reassuring the patient through personal attention. It is important to remember that hostility and guilt are the basic problems of the agitated depressed patient, and that their expression is to be accepted calmly and their stimulation to be avoided.

Physical needs. The maintenance of adequate nutrition for patients with aggressive patterns of behavior is essential and may present difficulty. Frequent small feedings of easily digested foods is often necessary because metabolism is either speeded up or slowed down. Eating should be carefully supervised to ensure an adequate intake, and weight should be checked at least once weekly. Careful attention to personal likes and dislikes in regard to food and attractive servings are usually worth the effort. The overactive patient's needs for extra caloric intake should be met. Fluid intake is neglected by patients with these disorder patterns, and a regular schedule for giving fluids, reinforced with easily digested caloric content, should be instituted and followed through.

Elimination is a constant problem, and every effort should be made to avoid a resort to cathartics since their administration so often presents a psychologic problem. Adequate fluid intake, regular toilet schedule, and adequate diet roughage should be employed routinely.

The problem of insomnia is ever present for the active patient because he is too busy to sleep and for the retarded and agitated depressed patient because he is too tense. Warm baths in preference to showers at bed time, allowance of adequate time to settle down, and use of as many physical measures as possible are indicated. Warm milk at bedtime, the reduction of stimuli, a high pillow, back rubs, and a comfortable bed are all measures of importance. Careful observation as to the actual hours of sleep should be given in order that measures may be taken to avoid exhaustion if necessary.

Personal cleanliness is the responsibility of personnel for any patient in an acute stage. The period of bathing should be utilized to promote personal relationships that are healthy, but special attention should also be given to care of the skin, hair, and nails and to oral hygiene. Physical condition and physical well-being are closely related to emotional responses, and the patient should be kept as physically comfortable as is possible in order to add no burden to his emotional problems. Personal appearance should be kept at the highest level possible because of its effect on the patient's self-opinion and on the response of others to him.

All patients in this group are careless in regard to personal appearance, personal cleanliness, and physical symptoms. Therefore, careful observation in regard to symptoms of physical illness is necessary. In addition, slow healing is characteristic so that prompt and efficient attention to infections and their treatment is essential.

It is interesting to note the close relationship between the physical status and clinical condition of patients with aggressive patterns of behavior. A loss of appetite and weight goes along with an increase in severity of symptoms, and an increase in weight and hours of sleep often presages clinical improvement. For this reason, if for no other, serious efforts to improve the general physical status of the patient are included in the general plan of treatment, and their importance cannot be minimized.

Protection. The protective needs of patients with aggressive behavior patterns are quite high. Exhaustion, injury to others, injury to self, and suicide are common enough occurrences to warrant constant alertness directed toward their prevention.

Exhaustion can be produced by overactivity, agitation, or tension. The physical condition of such patients should be carefully observed, and indications for intercession should be acted upon. The nurse should not be confused by the degree of output of energy as to the reserves the patient has left. Measures to avoid exhaustion are the limitation of activity by physical or chemical means, the careful avoidance of stimulation and irritation, the maintenance of fluid and caloric intake, and elimination. Accurate observation and reporting are essential.

Injury to others may occur through the impulsive gestures of overactive and aggressive patients or agitated and depressed patients. The danger is somewhat less in the instance of the retarded depressed patient, but not entirely absent while the patient is active enough to carry out a hostile gesture. Close observation and thorough knowledge of the patient's behavior patterns are aids in preventing such injuries. Recognition of mounting tension as indicated by voice changes, muscular signs of tensions, and increasing irritation are indications to take action to avoid possible injury to others. In addition, objects that can be used for assault should be restricted.

Self-injury short of suicide is fairly common in both overactive and agitated depressed patients. The former usually sustains injuries through impulsiveness and the latter through his agitated picking at himself. Alert observation, distraction, and occupation of the patient in some constructive activity are usually the best preventive measures. The care of injuries presents quite a problem because of the patient's lack of ability to assist in treatment. Therefore, prevention is the best measure.

The danger of suicide is quite marked in depressed patients and is present to some degree in overactive patients since flashes of their underlying depression are often seen. The single best precaution against suicide is an alert and imaginative nurse who is aware of all the patient's potentialities, aware of the possible methods open to the patient, and acutely sensitive as to how the patient actually feels. If such assurance is lacking, various measures may be used in a precautionary manner. A special close observation of the patient may be ordered, with responsibility specifically delegtaed to some one person at all times. A depressed patient is always a suicidal danger, and the nurse should ever be conscious of the fact that the patient's life may depend on her ability to observe him and understand how he feels. When caution to prevent suicide is being exercised, there is always the danger that concern for such prevention dominates thinking, feeling, and acting on the part of the personnel to the extent that other aspects of care become subordinated. Actually, suicide prevention is probably enhanced when other aspects of care, such as acceptance and attention to patients for purposes other than suicide prevention, are carried out faithfully.

With the agitated patient, the danger is always great. With the retarded patient the danger is most acute as he goes into and comes out of the depression. It is axiomatic that any patient who talks of death or suicide, who has feelings of guilt, who feels unworthy, who has no goal in life, or who is depressed is a potential suicide.

Group relations. The overactive, aggressive patient is far from being a total loss in a group. Unless there are too many like him, which can be extremely disruptive, he can be quite an asset. His values are derived from the fact that he can initiate activity, although he may not carry it through, and that he can simulate responses from withdrawn and retarded patients that a person in an authoritarian position may not be able to do. The danger to him lies in the fact that his domineering aggressiveness may draw group reaction against him, and his sensitivity may render him quite susceptible to hurt. Also, his aggressiveness may secure for him an undue amount of time and attention from personnel, which may result in a group united against him. If these precautions are kept in mind, his entrance in groups may be promoted, and assistance may be given him when he is in difficulty by distracting him from his course of action and substituting another that will bring peace for the moment. For him, that is all that is necesary since he is more or less at the mercy of environmental stimulation. The association with quiet patients may also tone him down somewhat since they are not particularly stimulating. If, however, their very quietness irritates him, contact with such patients should be minimized as far as possible.

The retarded depressed patient will isolate himself if possible, but should be encouraged to be with other patients even though he does not participate actively in a verbal sense or share too much in physical activities. The presence of others like himself is a little reassuring since it does not make him seem so alone and so different. Associations only with patients like himself would not result in any specific stimulation; therefore he should be exposed to more active patients. He should be allowed to advance to more shared activities at his own rate of speed since socialization is not quite the urgent necessity that it is for a patient with a withdrawal pattern. Depressions tend to self-limitation, and the period for more aggressive therapy is during their absence.

Agitated depressions also tend to be self-limited, and for patients in this group it is truly fortunate. They almost invariably irritate other patients and tend to be a source of group discontent. They may function to unite the group against them, which is not particularly good for the patient although it may be good for members of the group. The example of personnel attitude may help patients tolerate the agitated one. However, isolation from the group is more frequently indicated than in other types of illness. The prognosis for this particular behavior pattern is good; therefore, the acute phase may be handled in terms of the patient's ultimate recovery.

Convalescence. The convalescent period is one of return of responsibility to the patient for his own behavior and destiny. It is inevitable, and with this particular group of patients it involves a calculated risk. More patients actually succeed in committing suicide during the convalescent period than during the acute period, especially overactive aggressive and retarded depressed patients. The nurse must therefore be extremely alert and not in the least lulled into a false security by the patient's seemingly normality. She must always be accessible to the patient and encourage his free discussion of any topic with her in order to have an opportunity to assess his true emotional state. And she must be very tactful about it.

It is quite customary to see the patient go through a mild swing in the opposite direction from his illness, and the nurse should expect and be prepared for it. The overactive patient often has a mildly depressed period, and the depressed patient often has a mildly elated period. Signs of ominous significance during the convalescent stage are insomnia, loss of appetite or weight, and irritability. Another signal of significance is a sudden comfortable relaxation in the midst of obvious tension. Such occurrence usually indicates that the patient has made a decision, and a decision made under such conditions may be unwise even to the point of determination of a definite method of suicide.

Approaches to normal should be quietly encouraged. If the patient wishes to talk about his experience, well and good. Encourage it. Do not, however, embarrass a patient by talking about his acute period unless he indicates he wishes it. Even then, no judgment should ever be passed.

If the patient presents the opportunity, encouragement should be given him to utilize his better adjustment through continued psychotherapy. If the opportunity presents, the patient should also be encouraged to recognize signs in his own behavior that may indicate a relapse and need for a return to treatment.

References

Arieti, Silvana: Manic depressive psychoses. In Arieti, Silvana, editor: American handbook of psychiatry, New York, 1959, Basic Books, Inc., vol. 1, pp. 419-454.

Bigelow, Newton: The involutional psychoses. In Arieti, Silvana, editor: American handbook of psychiatry, New York, 1959, Basic Books, Inc., vol. 1, pp. 540-545.

Ewalt, Jack R. and Farnsworth, Dana L.: Textbook of psychiatry, New York, 1963, McGraw-Hill Book Co., pp. 188-206.

Fernandez, Theresa M.: How to deal with overt aggression, American Journal of Nursing 59:658, May 1959.

Noyes, Arthur P. and Kolb, Lawrence C.: Modern clinical psychiatry, ed. 6, Philadelphia, 1963, W. B. Saunders Co., pp. 305-323.

Rykken, Marjorie B.: The nurse's role in preventing suicide, Nursing Outlook 6:377-378, July 1958.

Schwartz, Morris S., and Shockley, Emmy Lanning: The nurse and the mental patient, New York, 1956, Russell Sage Foundation, pp. 21-71, 167-181.

Chapter XII

Nursing care of patients with projective patterns

In this group of personality disorders, the major mechanism of adjustment is denial and projection. Although the use of projection is liberally sprinkled throughout all forms of personality deviations, it is often simply a small part of another broad pattern of behavior. In some instances it dominates the disorder, and other mechanisms become subordinate to its use and tend to support the conclusions reached through projection. Some overlapping with the withdrawal pattern of deviate behavior exists; although even when this does happen, the patient tends to retain a better personality organization than is usually consistent with the extreme forms of withdrawal.

The projective disorders characteristically occur in middle-aged persons. This finding is consistent with a better retained personality organization since the patient has certainly managed to crystallize some adjustive techniques which have served to carry him well into adulthood.

Dynamics of development

A tendency to develop a suspicious attitude and projective techniques of adjustment is found in persons whose childhood produced hatred, chronic insecurity, suspiciousness, pride, inability to develop social skills, and a rigid, self-centered personality organization. Such a result is usually produced by a combination of factors in early experience. The child first develops a sensitivity to situations which made him feel inadequate and inferior, usually because this is his parents' perception of him. This feeling of inadequacy is reinforced by patterns of suspiciousness that are characteristic of the significant adults in his life. Also, usually rather extravagant demands are made on the child, and the standards of performance and conformity to which he is expected to adhere are unfortunately high. This overcompensatory insistence on status and prestige and on higher standards than others in the immediate environment, which reflects the parents' insecurity, produces several results in the child. It renders him sensitive to the opinions of others, and it strengthens narcissistic tendencies. It also arouses deep hostility which the child is afraid to express and must learn to hide.

The result is a person with a hostility-laden outlook, chronic insecurity, sensitivity, pride, and suspiciousness which make it extremely difficult for the growing personality to develop social skills in interpersonal relationships. A proud person finds it hard to talk problems over with others since it necessitates the admission to another that all is not well. The accompanying suspiciousness further checks any effort to establish satisfactory relationships with others. Brooding or introspective rumination becomes a fixed method for dealing with personal problems. Because of his inability to establish relationships with others, the individual finds it harder and harder to understand or appreciate any viewpoint except his own. As a result, reality testing becomes a lost art.

The personality organization becomes increasingly rigid as outside influence finds it more difficult to make an impression. Yet a sensitivity to outside opinions is retained, without the ability to evaluate it objectively.

Within the matrix of such a personality, which is unable to tolerate suspense, prolonged anxiety, or sustained tension, the projection of self-inadequacies and self-criticism to others follows readily. By this means, the basic hatred within the patient and his unacceptable impulses and wishes are denied as part of himself and projected to others around him, even if he has to invent some one as the object of projection. One's faults and failures are attributed to others and disclaimed for the self. The process not only produces comfort by ridding the self of unacceptable facets, but also makes one feel comfortably superior by comparison. It serves the purpose of avoiding loss of prestige or affection.

The ability to check this tendency by validating conclusions objectively against what has actually happened is defeated by the personality structure. When tension and anxiety are built up and are sustained, events are misinterpreted, and significance is attached to the environmental happenings that are in accord with the self-criticism and pride of the individual. Gradually the environmental forces are felt to be aligned in a plot or plan to harm the suspicious person. This offers at least an explanation for what is going on and gives some relief from doubt and suspense. Delusions of persecution have developed. Since the individual has been unable to develop techniques for retesting and analyzing situations in which he is personally involved and has arrived at the conclusion that he is persecuted, this conclusion is extremely difficult to change. Further inferences are made upon the basis of the assumption of persecution, and those parts of experience that support it or can be misinterpreted to support it are selected for attention. The delusional system becomes more or less systematized. Past events are recalled to support the assumption and distorted to confirm the delusions.

The rigidity and self-centeredness of the individual, along with his sensitivity and the almost inevitable gap between his demands on himself and his capacities, render him vulnerable to the use of projective patterns to defend himself in his own self-esteem. The projective pattern bolsters the ego since it both makes one important enough to be persecuted and gives a solid alibi for failure. If the anxiety and threat to security produced by the emotional response to the persecutory delusional system continues, delusions of grandeur may be the next resort. They may simply be a direct reaction to the self-criticism expressed in the original delusional system or they may result as an outgrowth of phantasied achievement with which the patient consoles himself.

Range of behavior

The degree to which projective methods of adjustment are used varies widely, and the behavior that results is a reflection of the degree. All of us behave to some extent on the assumption that other persons are as we are—that they share the same values, feelings, attitudes, and dislikes. The less experienced the individual, the more likely he is to act on this assumption in situations in which it is unwarranted. In addition, projection is more likely to operate in areas that involve socially forbidden and unacceptable actions. We ascribe to others motives of selfishness, evil intentions, and malice aforethought in behavior quite frequently although we are eager and anxious to disclaim any such motives on our own part. This is quite similar to the tendency of children to avoid punishment by denying bad behavior and placing responsibility on others or, if caught outright, to try to implicate others. When confronted suddenly with criticism or blame, the majority of adults will find some quick alibi that places blame on circumstances or persons other than themselves.

When a vulnerable, suspicious personality is exposed to prolonged tension and anxiety, it becomes necessary to protect self-esteem and projection is used as a bolster. The domination of the patient's behavior by delusional ideas is the point at which he usually shows a frank mental illness. One of the first symptoms to appear is rigidity of thought and loss of flexibility. The patient becomes unable to form correct judgments concerning events that occur. As the delusional ideas come to dominate the patient's behavior, the failure in judgment becomes apparent. The suspiciousness and brooding sensitivity become more marked, and ideas of reference follow in which the patient refers all happenings in his surroundings to himself and feels that everything that goes on has some special significance for him. Events are misinterpreted. Suddenly, things clear up. The patient realizes that a conspiracy against him is afoot. At first such false beliefs, or delusions, are fairly well organized, but they tend to spread, and the longer they exist, the more is woven into them, and the less logic there is to them. The Federal Bureau of Investigation is out to prove that the patient is a Communist; the world and all its environs are united against him. Ideas of influence then appear; that is, the patient feels his behavior is influenced by outside forces. Radar messages are transmitted to him that force him to commit acts against his will. Electric wires are attached to his brain, and derogatory messages are sent to him constantly. The patient's wife or husband, anxious to engage in an undisturbed extramarital affair, has had the innocent patient committed to the hospital and has planted nurses and attendants in the institution to make obscene remarks and drive the patient crazy. If perchance the patient is driven to take defensive or vengeful action toward his tormentors, counteraggression is automatically called forth, and this reinforces the patient's delusions.

Hallucinations may occur in the more serious manifestations. The patient hears voices accuse him of homosexual behavior or hears voices making threats against him. Grandiose delusions may make their appearance, and the patient believes he is Christ, Napoleon, or someone of stature between the two.

The emotional reaction to the psychotic behavior and ideas may range from completely adequate and appropriate to completely inadequate and inappropriate. The patient may feel a natural resentment against the forces aligned against him, may be mildly annoyed, or may discuss his delusional content with complete indifference. The adequacy of the emotional response is often fairly well correlated with the degree of logic or systematization of the delusions.

Nursing care

The unfortunate individual who isolates himself from sharing experiences with others is not a happy person, nor is he easy to reeducate. Persons for whom he reaches or who reach toward him are frustrated and thwarted by the reactions he calls forth, reactions which make friendship and warmth difficult under ordinary circumstances. The patient can admit no fault in himself and no virtue in others, a trait which is uncomfortably irritating until it is recognized that a fault in himself or a virtue in others threatens him seriously. His tendency to misinterpret situations and read into them derogatory motivations threatens the persons about him. Hence his nursing care is often more easily planned than carried out.

Psychotherapeutic environment. One of the basic ingredients of the psychotherapeutic environment must be a lack of counter-aggression or retaliation against the patient for his ideas because at this point the vicious circle can be broken. The patient's symptoms defeat his attempts to reach security and reasonable self-esteem because they call forth counteraggression which confirms the defensive need for the symptoms. The environment must reduce sharply the difference between the standards expected of the patient and his abilities. It must offend his sense of importance no more than is absolutely necessary. Activities must be available that offer some satisfaction, and the ward routine should have some intellectual challenge while being systematic enough to contribute to security. The environment should also offer the patient full opportunity to explore relationships and to explore such relationships within the limits of safety.

Interpersonal relationships. The very impersonality of a hospital and its routine offers the projectively inclined patient a sense of relief. It holds a reduction of the threat that more intimate relationships present. However although reduced, the threat remains implicit in the very presence of people. The patient's initial reaction to the hospital should be interpreted in this light.

The ultimate goal of interpersonal relationships with the patient is a contribution to his security in such relationships, a building of his sense of importance and prestige within the framework of reality, and a reduction of the demands he makes on himself. The patient's symptoms become obstacles in the path to this goal. This is the factor that has made it impossible for society to meet the patient's needs. The obstacles are a superior attitude, sarcasm and ridicule, extreme pride and sensitivity, overemphasis on status and prestige, an inability to see any other viewpoint, self-centeredness, misinterpretation of the behavior of others, and inflexibility. How are these to be met?

A superior attitude is invariably accompanied by the implication that all others are thereby inferior. Conceit, justified or otherwise, does not make for popularity because it makes other persons uncomfortable, places them on the defensive, and encourages attack and retaliation. It is important for the nurse to be able to recognize this response since she will most certainly feel it, and in the interest of the patient, she must control it. The superior attitude meets a deep-seated emotional need of the patient—it builds his self-esteem. To retaliate, to "teach the patient his place," makes certain that the patient will continue his behavior. Accept it and recognize its purpose. If the patient were as superior as his attitude indicates, he would not need the attitude. Contribute to his sense of importance constructively by praise for real ability and accomplishments and in the meantime let the patient pretend he is superman. He needs to.

Sarcasm and ridicule are used by the patient as a support for his superior attitude and his sense of importance. The purpose behind such behavior is to reduce the status of others and to make the patient appear better by comparison. Sarcasm and ridicule should be met with a matter-of-fact manner, and explanation, justification, and self-defense should be foregone. This again is not easy since few persons are so completely secure that they are comfortable under direct attack. However, since the patient needs the attitude and behavior, which spring from his basic self-doubt, it is important that the response to him contain no further challenge to his self-esteem.

The extreme pride and sensitivity of the patient make imaginative tact and courtesy necessary. Slights and offenses tend to be taken when none are meant. The particular points on which the patient is most sensitive should be learned and respected. Thoughtless comments and answers can cause a great deal of difficulty.

The patient's overemphasis on status and prestige may lead to certain problems in interpersonal relationships which can be difficult to handle. The patient may hold himself completely aloof from others and consider himself apart from and above everyone else, including personnel. He may identify with personnel an attempt to set up a pseudointimate relationship which places him above other patients in status. Such behavior should be quietly accepted, but if group retaliation against the patient is to be avoided, the patient should be tactfully guided into channels that involve participation in activities with other patients. It should be remembered that at the moment he is not an individual capable of tolerance for the weaknesses of others and therefore should not be turned loose on others who are acutely sensitive to open attack on their faults. On the other hand, the benefits of status and prestige should be conferred wherever possible for constructive accomplishments.

The tendency for the patient to misinterpret behavior in terms of his emotional needs should be recognized, and such misinterpretation should be assessed for its worth. If, for example, the patient is praised for three accomplishments and reprimanded for one mistake, the reprimand will receive more selective attention and be responded to more strongly than the praise. Such elements that lead to self-doubt should be avoided. When the patient does misinterpret, reason should not be used in order to change his mind. The misinterpretation is a symptom of illness, and for as long as the patient needs it, he should be permitted its indulgence. Only when negative emotions and behavior are calmly accepted by others does the sick patient have an opportunity to see them objectively himself.

The self-centeredness, inflexibility, and inability to see any other viewpoint must be recognized in their implications for nursing care. Reason is useless in their face until the patient has attained sufficient security to lose the need to be so rigid. Lengthy explanations and attempts to justify someone else's point of view are blocked and are therefore simply irritating to the patient. An approach which emphasizes altruistic motives, doing things for others, and having tolerance for others is doomed to defeat and simply makes the patient uncomfortable. In addition, such an approach demands something the patient cannot give and therefore increases his self-doubt.

The matter of how to respond to the psychotic ideas expressed by the patient is of paramount importance. That the entire personnel of the Federal Bureau of Investigation and the Secret Service are persecuting an innocent individual is rather absurd when checked against reality. The first step is to listen in full to the patient's expression without either agreeing or disagreeing. Answers to direct questions concerning the patient's psychotic content should be avoided unless the patient insists on a reply. Frequently many of the patient's questions are simply rhetoric, and if personnel do not interrupt the flow of conversation to answer questions, the patient goes on. Actually, the patient is much less interested in what other people think than in what he thinks and feels. Direct contradiction of the patient's ideas should be avoided, and they should not be brushed aside as nonsense. As a rule the patient has been shushed, called absurd, and reasoned with beyond endurance. Listen to him first and at length. Note carefully what is said and record it. During an acute phase, do no more than let the patient talk and avoid doing any talking about the patient's ideas if at all possible.

Hostility expressed in vengeful attack on the environment or persons in it should be controlled without punishing the patient for his behavior.

Physical needs. Because of his suspiciousness and his delusions of persecution, the patient frequently presents problems in the maintenance of nutrition. If he fears being poisoned, a careful study should be made of ways to get him to eat, up to and including indulgence of his rituals to make sure that his food is free from poison. Tube feeding should be avoided if at all possible because it is practically an invitation to the patient to misinterpret the procedure as counteraggression. If the patient's illness is chronic or of long standing, attention to the details of personal appearance and cleaniness may be the responsibility of personnel.

Protection. The protection of the projective patient centers, of course, around the symptoms he has developed to protect his ego. Since he sees himself as a person largely sinned against, he is always a potential danger to others because he may take action against what appears to him a vindictively hostile world. The patient should have adequate observation, and the possibility of attack on others should be guarded against. Two particular situations warrant special attention. If the patient retains a strong and appropriate emotional response to his psychotic ideas, retaliation on his part is more likely to occur. If, however, he recites his long list of persecutions without seeming to be disturbed by them, the danger is less. Projection against specific persons in the immediate environment is also an indication for alertness to possible danger. If the patient weaves the doctor, the nurse, the attendant, or another patient into his delusional system, the persecutor is handy for retaliatory action. In such an instance, the personnel member should be warned, or if a patient is involved, protection should be afforded him.

Early stages of the illness may be accompanied by depression, which is an indication of the danger of suicide. The patient may also react to his psychotic ideas with depression because he feels overwhelmed by an environment with which he cannot cope. In either instance, precautions against suicide should be taken.

If the belief of the patient that all is right with him and all is wrong with the rest of the world is remembered, it is easy to understand that his hospitalization is a cruel and unnecessary step against him, in his estimation. Personnel should be alerted to the fact that such patients present a real elopement threat. There is so much psychologic trauma involved in an elopement and forcible return to the hospital that an escape is well worth the effort of prevention. If it does occur and the patient is returned to the hospital, his feelings in regard to the matter should be spared at all costs.

Group relations. The patient who leans heavily on the mechanism of projection tends to be isolated emotionally from the group. If he is at all active, he is likely to be a mild trouble center because of his seeming sense of importance, his suspicion of the motives of others, and his intolerance for the faults of others. However, the relative impersonality of hospital personnel can be an extremely constructive experience for the patient and may lay the groundwork for the later establishment of closer relationships in the hospital group and in society.

The patient should be encouraged to work or play with other patients, starting with a limited number. Large groups either overwhelm him or afford him a screen behind which he can evade. Intellectual activities and detail work are usually his forte and should be permitted. Any activity that can be shared should be encouraged since skill in social relationships is a real need for this individual. He likes the importance of responsibility and may be allowed to help with slower and more withdrawn patients. In such situations the contribution to his own self-esteem may curb his expression of contempt for others. The appeal for such efforts should be directed to the patient's personal gain rather than to the benefits that will be derived by others. The projective patient cannot afford the luxury of altruism.

It may be necessary to protect other patients from this patient, but it is also necessary to realize that there are times when he himself may need protection. He can usually defend himself verbally against any onslaught, but the very act of defending himself indicates that his pride and sensitivity have been hurt. At such times he needs diversion from group activities and support. He should also be guarded against completely isolating himself and remaining aloof.

Convalescence. As the patient's behavior improves, it is not unusual for him to go through a long period during which he retains his psychotic ideas but does not let them govern his behavior so completely nor express them so freely. During this period, direct contradiction of the ideas he holds or admits having held is still not wise. Other explanations may be given for the patient to think about, but there should be no demands upon his acceptance of such explanations. If the patient insists upon an answer as to whether personnel believe his persecutory or grandiose ideas, a frank no may be given with the proviso that the patient is made aware that he has as much right to think yes as personnel have to think no.

Responsibility for himself will be returned to the patient, and any evidence of recrudescence of the illness should be carefully watched for as the time approaches for a return to society.

Social skills should be emphasized and encouraged during this period. The underlying sensitivity will probably always be a part of the patient; therefore development of social skills without making the patient uncomfortable will require unusual tact. This patient rarely experiences the sense of relief that a convalescing overactive or depressed patient does on escaping from the acute phase of his illness. He is very likely to be somewhat ashamed of his episode and to rationalize to justify it. Matter-of-factness toward mental illness on the part of personnel at this stage is very important to him. He may give the nurse little direct opportunity to demonstrate it in discussions with him, but he will be very alert as to how it is discussed with others in his hearing and as to how the nurse behaves toward mentally ill patients generally.

The patient in his convalescence needs as much support as can be given for realistic future plans. If he goes from the hospital retaining a wide discrepancy between what he expects of himself and what he is capable of accomplishing, he is vulnerable to a relapse. For that reason discussion of his future plans should be encouraged, which will give him an opportunity to see how they sound and to develop some objectivity toward them. Advice should not be given, and no decisions should be suggested. That the patient must be permitted to do for himself.

References

Cameron, Norman: Paranoid conditions and paranoia. In Arieti, Silvana, editor: American handbook of psychiatry, New York, 1959, Basic Books, Inc., vol. 1, pp. 508-539.

Cameron, Norman: The psychology of behavior disorders, Boston, 1947, Houghton Mifflin Co., pp. 427-445.

Noyes, Arthur P., and Kolb, Lawrence C.: Modern clinical psychiatry, ed. 6, Philadelphia, 1963, W. B. Saunders Co., pp. 367-378.

Stankiewicz, Barbara: Guides to nursing intervention in the projective patterns of suspicious patients, Perspectives in Psychiatric Care 2:39-45, 1964.

Sullivan, Harry Stack: Conceptions of modern psychiatry, Washington, D. C., 1947, William Alanson White Psychiatric Foundation, pp. 56-60.

Nursing care of patients who control anxiety with physical symptoms

C ommon to all persons whose illness falls within this group of personality disorders is a deep concentration on the physiologic aspect of existence as a method of avoiding anxiety and getting attention and approval. In such instances, no somatic basis for the difficulty can be demonstrated. A fatigue syndrome may occur without adequate physical explanation for its appearance, or such a morbid preoccupation with the state of health may occur that the entire routine of living is organized around the preoccupation. Actual physical symptoms, such as paralysis or anesthesia, may appear without somatic justification. In all such occurrences, the body and its function become a means of compromising with social demands. The method of adjustment rationalizes failure and brings a certain amount of sympathy from the persons in the environment, especially in the beginning of the particular ailment.

Dynamics of development

A constellation of early influences usually combines to produce a high degree of sensitivity to the normal function of the body and a deeper concern than is customary with physical health. Actually in our particular culture a certain attention is necessarily inculcated in all of us toward care and concern for the body. Since everyone learns early to note body changes, such as pain, and report them, generally a tendency develops to consider physiologic inadequacy a threat to security. A rather high degree of concern over physical status is normal to Western culture. In fact, only sin and sex can compete with constipation, weight, and physical illness as topics of conversation. When, however, solicitude over health or physical symptoms without an organic basis persists indefinitely in the face of contrary evidence and becomes a dominant factor in the pattern of living, then the point of normality has been transgressed.

In the development of such a behavior pattern, parental models are usually an important factor since children often adopt uncritically whole patterns of behavior from adults important to them without realizing or understanding what is happening. Fortunately for most of us, parents come in pairs, and one parent may counteract the destructive influence of the other. If the parents tend to share the same pattern, the likelihood of the child's adopting it is increased. Even if the child later, as a result of experiences outside the family, begins to drop a pattern so acquired, there remains the strong tendency to reactivate it in periods of stress and personal insecurity.

If the parents tend to be chronically anxious persons who respect and bestow attention upon fatigue, that is the pattern the child is likely to follow. If attention and increased affection are focused upon physical complaints and the parents use this type of behavior on the child, that is the pattern the child is likely to follow. If a great deal of attention is bestowed upon awareness of body function, that is the pattern the child is likely to follow. The use of fatigue and physical complaints unduly by the parents, or by the parent who has the greatest influence on the child, can predispose the growing personality to a similar defect in development.

Another form of behavior on the part of parents that tends to strengthen and overemphasize body concern is oversolicitude. The oversolicitude may be adopted as the child's own attitude toward himself, and, depending upon which particular type of body concern brings the greatest satisfactions, the groundwork for a fatigue syndrome, a morbid preoccupation with the state of health, or a definite physical disturbance may be laid.

Illness or injury during the early years or at times of stress may be the precipitating factor in overconcern with the body. This is particularly true if some degree of chronic insecurity is built into the personality structure. An individual, perhaps not too happy with himself and others, suddenly finds himself the center of attention, showered with sympathy, and reassured of his importance to others. It is a nice comfortable feeling, and the urge to experience it again can be very strong. When insecurity, anxiety, and tension mount again, the pattern of gaining reassurance and security through physical illness may be resorted to unconsciously. Repetition can build the habit firmly into the personality.

Extremely traumatic experiences, especially during early childhood, accompanied by severe anxiety can be instrumental in establishing the use of physiologic and pseudodisease processes as methods of adjustment. Strong emotions are accompanied by definite visceral changes which can be felt. It is not at all unusual for emotional disturbances that are severe to also be obscure in origin to the person affected. The art of repression can be employed here, and the individual reacts to the body sensations accompanying the emotional upheaval rather than to the cause. In fact the visceral changes may be perceived as the cause. The original precipitating factor in the emotional upset is pushed into the unconscious and cannot be brought to awareness. The anxiety produced is displaced onto the body processes in a sort of body protest. This happens most often in situations that are humilitating or dangerous. Such an experience or a succession of them may lead to overconcern with body function.

Add to any of these experiences a large element of credulity, and an interesting phenomenon in behavior may occur. An individual brought up in an atmosphere that is superstitious and uninformed is very likely to show hypersuggestibility and naivete that are rather unusual. Placed under severe stress or strain, he may show an unusual physical symptom that results in inactivation of some part of the body. This may be the unscientific stocking-and-glove anesthesia in which the anesthesia corresponds to the patient's ideas of the function of the part of the body and not to the actual nerve distribution. Other selective losses of function may occur, such as blindness, deafness, or inability to eat. The part involved is usually psychologically related to the anxiety-producing conflict, and the function of the illness, the control of anxiety, is often clearly hinted at by the patient's emotional calmness toward his symptom. This form of difficulty may be demonstrated also in episodic behavior disorders when seemingly an isolated behavior fragment takes over the personality temporarily. In such cases, multiple personalities and amnesias may be seen. The pattern just described is a rather naive one and is more commonly found in uninformed persons. Its incidence has been somewhat reduced by wide publicity.

All of these patterns serve common purposes. They either express anxiety or defend against it. In addition, they gain attention and interest and give the afflicted one a socially acceptable topic of conversation. Most of these patterns can, however, exhaust this effect as the persons around the patient eventually become annoyed, and rejection of the patient may finally occur. By this time the behavior pattern is so overlearned that it is difficult to change. The rejection increases the patient's tension and anxiety and leads to an accentuation of his behavior.

An element of compensation may enter the picture since the patient derives actual satisfaction from his behavior and the reception it gets. This can become a substitute satisfaction for the more usual ones the patient cannot achieve. One important factor in the pattern of body overconcern is that it supplies a rationalization for failures and inadequacies and has the advantage of being a socially acceptable one. Not so much is expected from the individual, and there is a ready excuse for failure to meet even moderate demands.

The same pattern can also be used aggressively to punish others. A paralyzed bedridden person can be a tyrant who rules the household with an iron rod. A husband who ventures a criticism of the management of the household finances can be brought in line with a severe headache that forces his wife to bed. He caused the headache, he misses his golf game, he cooks the supper, and he is kept busy carrying icecaps and reassurance to the bedside.

All of these techniques are part of an escape or evasion of the demands of one's self and of reality. They control anxiety and bring peace, but at a price. The price is the denial of a full, rich life.

Range of behavior

The range of behavior shown by persons with this particular group of disorders has already been indicated to some extent. The fatigue syndrome is one so closely related to normal that it is only under stringent criteria that it can be classified otherwise. Fatigue can be produced by overexertion or by lack of rest and is a common experience. The degree of resistance also varies from time to time in individuals, and the fluctuation is often a measure of interest in the task to be done. When fatigue appears consistently too readily, when it is out of all proportion to the exertion involved, when it impairs social effectiveness over a prolonged period, or when an individual's life becomes organized around fatigue, the behavior is deviating from the range of normal.

The usual presenting complaint is a feeling of exhaustion, of being utterly worn-out. The slightest exertion produces weakness and wanness, and it is necessary to plan routines and activities that are restricted to a mild output of energy. Secondary symptoms usually occur, including headaches, heightened sensitivity to any sensory stimulation, discouragement, irritability, and difficulty in remembering or concentrating. This is a picture that we can identify in ourselves at one time or another.

The personality disorders centered around physiologic functions and complaints related to them are extremely varied in manifestation and may involve almost any part of the anatomy. The gastrointestinal tract probably leads all others in incidence of involvement. This is reasonable since early habit training involves a great deal of emphasis on the processes of eating and elimination. Strong cultural attitudes, taboos, and rituals continue to be associated with the use of both ends of the alimentary tract throughout life. In addition, the function of the gastrointestinal tract is easily observed, is open to some degree of control, and is an acceptable topic of social conversation. The actual range of complaints that lead the patient to a doctor may involve any part or all of the system and include the following: heartburn, indigestion, nervous stomach, pains related to the eating period, diarrhea, constipation, inability to eat, and so forth, ad infinitum. The actual task of distinguishing between the use of such complaints as a method of behavior adjustment and actual gastrointestinal disease is not always easy.

Other systems frequently involved are the cardiovascular, the respiratory, the genitourinary, and the neuromuscular. The symptoms of almost any disease of these systems can be the presenting complaint of the patient, and not too seldom the pattern of complaints fits no particular illness. In each instance, careful evaluation of the actual physical status of the patient is necessary to rule out somatic disease. Related to the cardiovascular system, among the commonest symptoms are rapid pulse, palpitation, breathlessness, pain, dizziness or faintness, and throbbing blood vessels. Many of them can be symptoms of actual cardiovascular disease, but many of them can also be the visceral expression of strong emotional responses. The genitourinary tract is used more often by women in a neurotic adjustment, probably because of the menstrual cycle, the more dramatic climacteric, and the incidence of serious gynecological diseases among women.

The particular organ or system around which the patient organizes his life is largely a matter of personal experience. Any symptom or combinations of symptoms found in a medical textbook can be duplicated by such patients, plus many combinations not found in any textbook. Generally speaking, the better informed the public is in relation to the function of an organ or system, the more closely will the patient's syndrome approximate a real disease. With this particular reaction pattern, the patient usually worries a great deal about his complaints and is openly and deeply concerned about them.

Another group of physical symptoms without adequate organic basis is characterized by a selective loss of function or normal activity and is usually accepted by the patient with a calm emotional attitude. Several of the commoner types will be described as illustrations. In many instances, the loss of function or activity would seem to the lay person to be due to neurologic damage or disease.

The partial or complete loss of the ability to speak is a common occurrence in normal stress situations, such as a sudden shock, fright, or the receipt of bad news. A precipitating situation of the same nature may produce speechlessness in a susceptible personality in which the symptom persists because of anxiety or some unmet need. The physical structures involved continue to function well except for speaking.

A partial or complete loss of appetite is also common in excitement, anger, or conflict. The process of eating is one with strong social implications since taking food is usually an experience shared with others and generally means some degree of social acceptance or at least tolerance. It is often a symbolic process indicating acceptance by a chosen group, as in the ritual of communion in the Christian religion. The loss of the ability to eat in emotional disorders is usually related to the symbolic significance of eating and is a form of rejection or isolation by the patient. The recovery from this particular form of disorder is not usually dramatic since, once the patient does begin to eat, it requires some time to rebuild the body tissues.

The loss of specific motor activities and the loss of response to sensory skin stimulations are ordinary experiences. People get frightened "stiff" or "paralyzed" by danger. Ordinarily painful stimuli may not be felt under such circumstances. In a fist fight or in battle, injuries are often sustained that are not felt or realized until the period of immediate danger or fright has ended. When loss of motor activity becomes a major facet of existence, without organic cause for the loss, pathologic behavior is then evidenced. Paralysis may occur in any part of the body—legs, arms, shoulders, or lower half of the body. The distribution of the paralysis may not be neurologically justified, and the loss of activity may relate to only one function. For example, the patient may not be able to walk, but may be able to move his legs about quite normally while in bed. The development of secondary contractures and atrophies may occur if the paralysis persists. Anesthesias which also occur usually have a sharp boundary line and tend to follow lay ideas of functional anatomy. There is no response to painful stimulation in the hand, the arms as far as the elbow, or the leg as far as the knee. In both anesthesias and paralyses, inconsistencies and contradictions in symptoms usually rule out damage to the nervous system as a causative factor.

A symptom which is particularly likely to show striking inconsistencies is the partial loss or complete loss of response to visual stimulation. Interference with vision sometimes occurs in anxiety or emotional tension although one result of anxiety may be to increase visual acuity. A more closely related normal phenomenon is the ability to inactivate the function of one eye and exclude its response to stimulation while using the other eye to concentrate on a specimen under a microscope. The degree of loss of vision may vary widely. The sudden, miraculous recovery of sight that is headlined in newspapers now and then is frequently open to suspicion that the person has one of these personality disorders.

Another interesting loss of function, and one that is usually considered newsworthy, is the partial or complete loss of the ability to respond to stimulation leading to recall or recognition. This loss of memory, or amnesia, may vary in degree from forgetting a few incidents or parts of them through to forgetting whole episodes of one's life. Actually, it is much more common for incidents or episodes to be forgotten, without loss of self-identification. The latter does occur, however, and the patient cannot identify himself. Such episodes are exaggerations of the very normal tendency to forget the names of people we do not like, to forget more easily unpleasant experiences, and to leave personal articles at a place to which we wish to return.

Closely related to this latter group of personality disorders is a series in which isolated behavior fragments or episodes appear in an inappropriate environmental context or in opposition to the person's previous behavior pattern. These occur as motor activities of varying degrees of complexity. Tremors, which occur normally in periods of stress or physical weakness, can persist indefinitely and be of pathologic nature. Tics, or sudden involuntary muscle jerking, may occur and may involve only a small group of muscles or may be an elaborate affair involving a considerable portion of the body. All of these are usually not accompanied by any serious disturbance in the patient's orientation. Other types may cause a complete but temporary break with the continuity of behavior, such as a seizure or convulsion. The pattern of the convulsion is usually the same for each patient, but may vary considerably from patient to patient.

The most complex disturbance in motor activity is the occurrence of a multiple personality in which two or more organized systems of behavior alternate in control of the individual, and each system remains unaware of the other or others. This is the ultimate in dissociation. Actually, it is comparatively rare to find patients with clear-cut alternating personalities. More likely to be found is the patient in whom there is a dominant personality system with fragmentary subsystems toward which the dominant is amnesic, that is, is not aware of their existence. The fragmentary system, which takes control of behavior on sporadic occasions, is aware of the actvities of the dominant system. This subordinate system is usually childishly immature.

Nursing care

No more misunderstood or maligned group of patients exists than those with physical symptoms and inadequate somatic pathologic conditions as an alibi. They are seldom found in psychiatric hospitals, but are more likely to fill the wards of general hospitals. They are not forgotten—they are disliked, abused, and the object of contempt and ridicule. Psychoneurotic behavior is acceptable only when it is one's own.

Psychotherapeutic environment. The reeducation of a patient overly concerned with the physical aspect of existence is best promoted in an environment in which the particular needs of neurotic patients can be met without too great a price to others. It is this factor that tends to defeat, under ordinary social conditions, the learning of new skills by hypochondriacal and hysterical patients. Removal from the immediate environment, including close contact with significant persons, is frequently indicated to reduce the pressure on the patient. In a more closely controlled environment, the reduction of demands on the patient is helpful. The pattern of evasion is deeply rooted, thoroughly overlearned, and clung to by the patient even when the behavior pattern defeats its own ends. Environmental adjustments are frequently necessary to make it possible for the patient to learn new methods of behavior.

The environment should also be one in which physical illness is not the center of attention and emphasis. Yet facilities should be available for a complete physical examination in order to rule out organic pathology and to have available the negative results of such an examination to reassure the patient once rapport has been established.

Two other factors are important in a psychotherapeutic environment—there should be a routine that permits a balance of work and play, since the recreational needs of neurotic patients tend to be high, and there should be enough pressure of activities to prevent the patient's being too much alone.

This would indicate that a general hospital ward may not be the ideal place for the treatment of personality disorders centered around the physiologic aspect of existence. Certainly the general hospital can be effectively used for a thorough physical examination in the initial stages of treatment, but the whole atmosphere and function of such a unit tends to be a handicap in helping the patient to learn new patterns of behavior.

Interpersonal relationships. The greatest single problem in the establishment of healthy interpersonal relationships with the neurotic group of patients is the recognition and control of the emotional attitude of personnel toward them. The patient is most commonly viewed as someone who is deliberately malingering and who is perfectly capable of behaving himself if he desires. Frequent comments, such as "There is *nothing* wrong with him," and "I can't be neurotic because I have a real pain," reveal the common fallacy in the thinking on neurotic disorders. True, there may be nothing physically wrong with the patient at the moment, but there is definitely something wrong—*the patient is sick!* In addition, surprising as it may seem, the neurotic pain is both real and severe. The patient feels it as much as though actual pathologic disease of tissue structures were present. To confront the patient with the fact that there is no organic reason for the pain or difficulty does not end the pain. It will continue to exist as long as the patient emotionally needs it. And it is *real* pain.

The ability to emotionally accept the fact that neurotic patients are truly sick, cannot themselves understand the relationship between their symptoms and their emotional problems, and are actually as physically uncomfortable as they say they are is essential for personnel who wish to help them. This tends to be one of the biggest stumbling blocks in the treatment of such patients since the members of the health team have usually thoroughly overlearned an organic approach to illness and have a mildly Spartan philosophy against which they tend to judge patients. The usual definition of a good patient by the persons who care for him is one who can take anything without complaint. This attitude should be brought out into the open and talked through with someone with a thorough understanding of such disorders the moment one finds he is being critical and contemptuous toward patients with physical symptoms that do not correlate with organic pathology.

The greatest technical problem in interpersonal relationships is conveying acceptance and a feeling of worth to the patient without emphasizing or paying undue attention to his physical complaints. It is usually wise early in contact with the patient to listen completely and intently to his description of his complaints and their history. As a rule, it has been a long time since anyone has listened to him patiently. Comments pro or con in regard to complaints should be avoided, and the listening should be done matter-of-factly but with interest. It is easier to avoid commenting than it would seem, for most patients are anxious to pour out their complaints, and they are not too interested in what someone else may think of them. If comments are necessary, they can be limited to repeating the feelings expressed by the patient such as discomfort, fear, anxiety, and worry. After one has listened through, it is then wise to avoid leading the patient into a discussion of his physical symptoms if possible. Diversion toward topics which interest the patient should be tried at every opportunity. When later or changing complaints are brought forth, they should be accepted calmly and relayed to the physician for evaluation. The appearance of excitement or contempt in regard to symptoms should be carefully avoided. Difficult though it may be from the emotional point of view, it is very important to seek out this patient when immediate routine and procedures do not demand it. It is one of the better ways of convincing the patient that he is a person of some worth.

Early in the patient's experience his pattern of behavior was helped toward fixation by the secondary gain he derived from his illness. This gain is the sympathy received for the presence of the symptoms themselves. While the patient is under treatment, this gain should not be reinforced. Calm acceptance of the patient's complaints and his right to them, without indicating by word or attitude any feeling of pity or of being sorry for him, is the best procedure. Accept the patient as a person without sanctioning his particular form of maladjustment.

Care in discussing medical knowledge with the patient or in his hearing should be exercised. These patients tend toward suggestibility and are wont to pick up new knowledge and weave it into the pattern of complaints. Questions asked in regard to specific symptoms of the patient should be limited since they may plant ideas of what else might be expected.

Neurotic patients also have a tendency to play personnel off against each other and usually attempt to discredit anyone who implies by word or look that their illness is not organic in nature. Personnel should avoid being caught in the process by being alert to its appearance.

Reassurance and encouragement should be given the patient carefully and not in relation to physical symptoms if it can be avoided. Positive accomplishments in other areas should be recognized and rewarded, particularly in the ability to develop recreational skills and to participate in activities with others.

Under present conditions, the majority of such patients will be found in general hospitals. The nurse should be able to recognize them and to understand both what she can do and what she cannot do for them. In the first place, she is not likely to cure or alter the course of events much for the patient unless she can be instrumental in guiding him toward psychiatric treatment. This suggestion may best be planted with receptive relatives if there are such. A great deal will depend upon the patient's physician and his attitude toward the patient's illness. The one constructive thing the nurse can do is give the patient intelligent nursing care during his hospitalization by understanding that his behavior, however annoying it may be, is an expression of his anxiety and self-doubt. If she can reassure the patient as to his worth through her own behavior and leave him feeling understood and comfortable with her, she has accomplished a good deal.

Physical needs. Generally, the physical needs of neurotic patients should be de-emphasized. However, since gastrointestinal complaints are so frequent, problems in regard to nutrition and elimination are fairly frequent. Attention to them should be tactful and almost surreptitious, and they should never be permitted to become a major issue in relations with the patient.

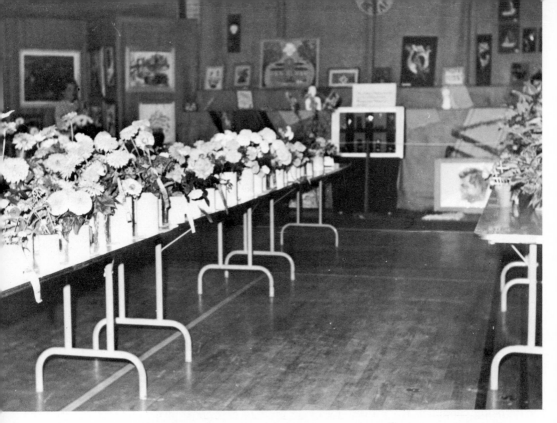

Patients take pride in entering flowers they have raised in a local flower show.

A good routine embodying sound health habits should be carried out, but this also should be done unobtrusively. The neurotic patient needs to learn to balance his life away from his concern with his body and its function.

Protection. Suicide and attacks on others are comparatively rare with neurotic patients although suicidal attempts resulting from unbearable anxiety over a prolonged period of time have occurred. The great protective need of these patients is from panic attacks which can be precipitated by mounting anxiety. The patient's behavior pattern becomes completely disorganized under overwhelming terror. In such a state, injury to self or others is quite possible. Another caution signal is constant verbalization about death or dying. Tactful precautions should always be taken if the patient shows any such preoccupation.

Panic can be avoided by reducing the patient's anxiety and by being careful not to cause the patient further anxiety. A study of the types of situations that tend to increase the patient's tension should be made, and such situations should be avoided if possible. Mounting tension and anxiety should be reported in order that preventive measures may be taken. The patient also needs to be protected from the development of a passive dependence on persons in the environment. Trends in this direction in interpersonal relationships should not be encouraged, no matter how flattering they may be.

Group relations. Neurotic patients, when first introduced into a group, tend to be accepted and sympathized with, but usually wear out their welcome rapidly and wind up being rejected. Patients on the whole accept them better than personnel. An early and consistent effort to keep them in the group and participating in shared activities often pays dividends. One or two other patients with similar problems can be a help since it gives the patient an opportunity to form with them a subgroup, with a sense of sharing, while remaining a part of a larger group. Isolation from the group should be avoided at all costs. Being alone too much grants many opportunities for concentration on body function.

Convalescence. During the period of convalescence, a very matter-of-fact de-emphasis of physical needs and body function should continue. The patient should be very tactfully supervised during routine to prevent fatigue since its symptoms may increase his interest in his body. The use of such procedures as enemas or sedation should be avoided, and all possible measures should be taken to prevent their use. As the time for discharge nears, a brief exacerbation of physical complaints may be expected and should be taken calmly, without indicating to the patient any anxiety over their appearance.

Social activites, particularly recreational, should be encouraged. Neurotic patients need to learn to play and to enjoy it, and the convalescent period is usually the best opportunity to promote this phase of the patient's treatment.

If the patient wishes to discuss or talk about his illness, he can be permitted to do so. Every care should be taken to show and to encourage the patient to show a healthy attitude toward mental illness. The patient will often need the support of interest in him and his activities while he remains somewhat awkward in his attempts to seek expression of such interest. No attention should be directed toward the patient's awkwardness in interpersonal gestures, but the interest should be expressed freely and without demands attached to it.

References

Abse, Wilfred: Hysteria. In Arieti, Silvana, editor: American handbook of psychiatry, New York, 1959, Basic Books, Inc., vol. 1, pp. 272-292.

Cameron, Norman: The psychology of behavior disorders, New York, 1947, Houghton Mifflin Co., pp. 187-277, 318-387.

Chrzanowski, Gerard: Neurasthenia and hypochondriasis. In Arieti, Silvana, editor: American handbook of psychiatry, New York, 1959, Basic Books, Inc., vol. 1, pp. 258-271.

Noyes, Arthur P., and Kolb, Lawrence C.: Modern clinical psychiatry, ed. 6, Philadelphia, 1963, W. B. Saunders Co., pp. 379-442.

Horney, Karen: Neurosis and human growth, New York, 1950, W. W. Norton & Co., Inc.

Schwartz, Morris S., and Shockley, Emmy Lanning: The nurse and the mental patient, New York, 1956, Russell Sage Foundation, pp. 182-198.

Sullivan, Harry Stack: Conceptions of modern psychiatry, Washington, D. C., 1947, William Alanson White Psychiatric Foundation, pp. 54-59.

Chapter XIV

Nursing care of patients who control anxiety through ritualistic patterns

Ritual, repetition, and magic play a considerable role in modern existence despite the emphasis on change in the social milieu that is so often stressed. Inflexibility in procedure is a common characteristic of children's play and story telling activities. Adults also have their rituals in religion, in organizations, and is personal daily routines. Most adults still cherish the magic illusion that a verbal apology wipes out the effects of past behavior and avoids possible consequences. The special virtue of ritual is the uniformity and sameness which is in effect a sort of control of the environment and self in that the ritual, performed always the same way, reduces any necessity for a decision and guarantees to some extent the results that follow. This type of behavior, found extensively in normal persons, can become exaggerated to an abnormal degree and can become so marked that it actually interferes with social effectiveness. When an irresistible impulse to say, do, or think some one thing seriously complicates existence and interferes markedly with an adjustment, then behavior is pathologically compulsive.

Dynamics of development

Compulsive behavior, characterized by mounting tension that is temporarily discharged by an indulgence in the compulsive act or thought, is closely related to the development of the techniques of self-control in the growing individual. Self-control is a social skill that follows a certain broad pattern of development. Discipline and correction are accomplished in the beginning through outside compulsion, which is brought about by the attachment of unpleasant experience to disapproved acts and by the attachment of pleasure and acceptance to acts that are approved. Eventually, the child accepts the responsibility for meeting approved standards on his own, in keeping with the values of his parents. This shift of responsibility occurs gradually, and the period of change is marked by ambivalence. The child both reaches for forbidden fruit and chastises himself for his desires and behavior. Emotional experience in the formative years of life that tends to prevent growth beyond the ambivalent period in conscience development provides fruitful soil for compulsive behavior.

Factors that are important in the early years are naturally related closely to parental patterns of behavior. Compulsive parents tend toward the production of compulsive children since children so frequently incorporate whole patterns of their parents' behavior. In addition, compulsive parents may carefully train their children in compulsive habits. If the children's compulsiveness is insisted upon as a condition of affection or acceptance, the habit will be a difficult one to dislodge in later years. Parents who are not themselves compulsive may also train their children in compulsive habits, especially if they are desirous of having offspring about whom they can brag inordinately to neighbors and relatives. Too much emphasis upon detailed procedure and precise end results can establish compulsive habits of work, and such patterns, learned in one type of situation and associated with approval, tend to spread to other areas of behavior. Interestingly enough, such methods of education were typical of schools of nursing of the immediate past. The procedure was the thing that mattered—the exactness in steps and the precise end result. Understanding of the whys in any given procedure went unmentioned. The precise end result now represents a profession still peopled with members who heatedly and unintelligently insist that the "way we gave a douche in my school of nursing is the *only* right way to do it!"

In addition to overemphasis upon procedure and precise end results, other parental dictates that are conducive to the development of compulsiveness are burdening children with too heavy a sense of responsibility too early and inculcating too much dread of mistakes and fear of retaliation. Training in guilty attitudes has a marked effect on personality structure. Impressing children with the retribution due immoral conduct long before they are able to understand immorality or ethical problems makes them prone to guilt reactions and confusion about their own thoughts and behavior. When behavior is shared with others, this early training may be overcome, but in all families and in all cultures there are taboos that will continue to produce guilt and conflict when one is trained in guilty attitudes. Relevant to this is our own cultural attitude toward sex. The average individual reaches adulthood having learned far more about sex guilt than sexual function or intelligent sexual self-control.

Parental handling of criticism can also be significant in the development of compulsive behavior. The stern and unforgiving parent who withholds affection at the child's slightest deviation from the path laid down for him can easily develop a submissive child who adopts as a ritual the performance that once or twice secures the affection he needs. Children, generally speaking, cannot tolerate rejection. A parent who is stern and exactingly demanding of the child builds attitudes of guilt and anxiety that may require ritualistic behavior to overcome.

Early experience and parental attitudes or examples may develop severe anxiety and overmeticulousness in a child. Such a child, constantly threatened by loss of affection over small details and relatively insignificant happenings, needs more than average reassurance and certainty. Security is constantly threatened, and *absolute* security becomes one of the child's emotional needs. By no stretch of imagination is it possible to achieve absolute security in modern existence. The adoption of ritualistic behavior under such circumstances limits free choice of action and serves several purposes. It reduces the number of experiences to which the individual must respond and reduces thereby the number of potential anxieties he must face; its sameness produces a certain form of security, and it becomes a defensive method of self-control. Actually, as an adjustive technique, it is not too successful. The anxiety that is discharged through compulsive behavior is only a transient relief since the anxiety builds up again and the compulsion must be indulged again. Such behavior also restricts experience and growth since one function of compulsions and rituals is to limit the range of experience to which the individual is exposed.

(impossible)

Types of behavior

The forms that compulsive behavior may take all have in common the irresistible urge to do, say, or think some one thing which the individual usually resists, with mounting anxiety, and then indulges with temporary relief from the anxiety.

The compulsion may involve repetition of some significant act or thought. The classic example is compulsive hand washing and is a performance that is easy to relate to the underlying guilt, the anxiety it produces, and the necessity to expiate it. In a culture in which cleanliness is next to godliness (and may even precede it!), the connection between cleanliness and lack of guilt is easy to grasp. The patient washes his hands frequently and becomes markedly anxious if the process is blocked. Some patients go through elaborate rituals to keep their hands clean and must wash them every time they come in contact with any object. For others, only some one object or types of objects may be the sources of contamination. Other acts, of course, may be repeated much in the same fashion as a dog must circle a spot several times before he can lie there comfortably. Practically any form of behavior can be involved. The return to the household that *must* be made to ascertain that cigarettes are out or that the gas is turned off are fairly normal examples.

The performance of a procedure in an exact order is another form of compulsion. This too can take practically any form that behavior takes. The patient who must dress in exact order is an example. He puts on the right sock, right shoe, left sock, and left shoe and then his coat; if he is not sure that this order was followed, he must undress and start all over to be sure. When the serial order of an act is so rigidly fixed that any slight deviation produces anxiety and requires the act to be done over from the start, the patient is then behaving compulsively. Such behavior requires the close attention of the patient and can absorb practically the whole of his waking time. Such behavior, severe enough, precludes any possibility of holding an ordinary job or carrying on a relatively normal existence.

Another form of compulsive behavior is compulsive orderliness or cleanliness. The average housewife who has this trait to a fairly marked degree usually has an enviable reputation as a "good wife and mother" in the neighborhood, a reputation which those who have to live with her would be likely to challenge. A meticulously kept house with a place for everything and everything in its place at all times is usually not a comfortable house in which to live. The significant fact in such orderliness or cleanliness that marks it as pathologic is the anxiety and inexplicably strong emotional reaction that any deviation produces.

Self-restraint and asceticism can be compulsive in nature when an individual keeps a rigid and unrelenting iron hand on himself and, all too frequently, on other persons. Rigid rules for conduct and severe penalties for mild infractions are common occurrences in such people. If they have children, the danger of development in a compulsive direction is rather above average for those children. Such persons are markedly perfectionistic, with an attention to details and minutiae that makes them a source of severe annoyance to those who must work with or under them.

The indulgence in superstition and magic beliefs and rituals can also become compulsive in nature. Actually, in the lives of all of us, no matter how scientific and intellectual, there are personal attitudes and beliefs that are influenced not at all by reason. Most of us have some superstitions and prejudices and magic beliefs that we keep hidden lest we be rediculed. Magic rituals that produce a marked anxiety when they are interfered with are compulsive. A patient's dependence upon magic procedures to allay anxiety can be pathologic. The person who becomes panic-stricken when he walks under a ladder, or who is "scared stiff" when a black cat crosses the street in front of him is actually not so far from normal—but he is off the path.

Antisocial compulsions are more common than one would expect, and the epitome of this form of behavior is the urge to kill another person. Although this appears most frequently as a phantasy of doing violence to others that is followed by deep feelings of guilt, it may carry over into overt action. A more commonly seen form of behavior is compulsive stealing—stealing that appears rather senseless on the surface. The patient usually steals articles for which he has no use or desire, does so only after tension and anxiety have built up, and experiences relief from anxiety when the theft is completed. A milder form, closer to a normal manifestation, is the irresistible urge to shock others verbally with obscene or vulgar comments. Allied to this are a whole group of sexual aberrations, such as sexual peeping or indecent exposure.

Another form of compulsive behavior is the obsessive fear, or phobia. The type of fear, such as fear of heights, darkness, crowds, or closed spaces, is usually related to the patient's past experience. All phobias have in common deep-seated fear of some object or situation which the patient himself cannot explain, and which produces panic if the patient is forced into the situation he fears.

Nursing care

Ritualistic patients present a difficult therapeutic problem. The long-standing need for absolute security and certainty makes any definite planning for them long range in nature. The restricting effect of their ritual upon their range of experience poses problems in dealing with the symptom itself in such a manner as to meet the patient's basic needs.

Psychotherapeutic environment. The basic essential in a psychotherapeutic environment for compulsive patients is a place where the patient is not handicapped or punished for his symptoms. To carry out the compulsive act itself is an absolute necessity for the patient during his illness since it does give transient relief from an anxiety that would otherwise overwhelm him. An environment so adjusted that the patient is not isolated or made conspicuous by the indulgence of his symptoms provides an important element in his treatment.

One of the purposes of ritualistic behavior is to relieve the patient of the necessity for making decisions. Therefore, the environment should be sufficiently controlled and routine consistent enough to tactfully relieve the patient of as many decisions as possible. The consistency in environment and routine also helps to limit the range of experience to which the patient is exposed. New experience carries a threat and should be carefully introduced.

The demands made upon the patient in regard to complying with routine and participating in activities should make full allowance for his anxiety, his ritual, and his unrecognized fear of experience that is new. In other words, the patient needs an environment in which he can be comfortably sick.

Interpersonal relationships. Interpersonal relationships are tools designed to contribute to the ritualistic patient's security, to the reduction of his anxiety, and to the building of his confidence in relations with others. The major problems presented by the patient's behavior are his ritualistic activity, his periodic mounting anxiety, his ambivalent attitude, his tendency to integrate situations that produce guilt, and his hostility that he fears to express except symbolically.

The compulsive act must be accepted in a comparatively permissive manner. When possible, its indulgence should be permitted in as constructive a manner as possible for the patient. For example, one patient relieved some degree of her anxiety by thoroughly scrubbing the shower stall after having her shower. When the activity was denied her, she became restless and anxious and was unable to carry on with the day's activities. Routine was adjusted for her so that she took her shower early in the day, scrubbed the shower stall thoroughly immediately thereafter, and was then able to join the patient group in recreational and occupational therapy. Because the completion of the compulsive act is usually succeeded by a feeling of relief, this period can be used consistently to treat any possible effects of the compulsive acts. In this instance, the problem was the prevention of damage to the skin on the patient's hands which tended to break down after the vigorous daily scrubbing with strong soap.

Ritualistic behavior is time consuming, and the patient must be allowed adequate time without any sense of pressure or criticism. Attempts to reason with the patient concerning his behavior are useless and will not influence the course of events except destructively. An intellectual explanation leaves the patient with a feeling of inadequacy and of having been criticized for his failure to meet the standards that are implied for him. The end result is an increase in anxiety and further guilt feelings for his failure. Extreme care must be observed in the attitude of personnel toward the symptom—it should be treated as though it were a completely natural and expected phenomenon. Any hint of criticism, any special attention, or any punitive measures must be carefully avoided in relation to the compulsive act.

When limits must be drawn on carrying out the compulsive act, as in serious interference with maintenance of the patient's health, the limits must be consistently enforced. In addition, the decision as to where the line is to be drawn should be determined for the patient and any necessary procedures, such as tube feeding, should be carried through quickly and efficiently. Long explanations and coaxing are usually upsetting and increase the psychologic trauma involved.

The patient's anxiety stems from confusingly ambivalent feelings and a deep sense of guilt. Helping the patient control anxiety involves taking full account of these important feelings. A great deal of patience and tact are necessary to avoid any comments or any hint of impatience in attitude or behavior that might increase the patient's sense of failure and his feeling of guilt. For this reason, discussion of the patient's symptom or symptoms should be only on his initiative. Any judgment in regard to the ritual must be scrupulously avoided. Every effort should be directed toward making the patient as thoroughly comfortable with and about his ritual as is possible.

An ambivalent attitude should be expected and calmly accepted. Alertness for its expression helps one to avoid reacting to ambivalence in a manner that may imply criticism of negative emotional expressions or undue praise of positive expressions. Dislike and hostility may be expected, even though they are not often too openly expressed. More positive emotions may be expressed at the same time or later. In either case, it is wise not to lean too strongly on the positive emotional expression or expect it to continue indefinitely. An attitude expressing approval of such behavior is a threat to the patient since he is incapable of maintaining the more positive level.

Since therapeutic interpersonal relationships must take account of the patient's reduced and restricted abilities, it is important with ritualistic patients to keep routine and attitudes as consistent as possible. New procedures and variety in established ones carry more threat than stimulation of interest and should be avoided. The pathologic need for absolute certainty should be respected, and every effort should be made to keep the patient as certain as possible about what to expect under any and all circumstances.

Many patients who rely on excessive ritualism show what, for lack of a better term, may be called verbal insight. They are, in the course of their illness, able to express some intellectual understanding of the relationship of their behavior to their feelings of guilt although they may be unable to indicate why they feel guilty. It should be recognized that it is very late in the course of treatment before this insight is accepted emotionally so that the patient is able to use his knowledge to influence his behavior. Insight of an intellectual nature that does not influence behavior is partial insight and is extremely painful to the patient. In a sense, he knows enough to be aware that he should be able to control his behavior, but he cannot. The result of such partial insight is to increase the patient's dissatisfaction with himself and to increase his sense of failure. Any expression of such verbal insight should be evaluated as to how it makes the patient feel about himself, and care should be taken in responding not to increase the patient's discomfort. Whenever such verbalization occurs while the patient continues his compulsive act, personnel should not be confused by what the patient has to say. Above all, they must not act as though they expected the patient to behave in conformity with the knowledge his words would seem to indicate.

Regardless of the particular problem, a carefully planned schedule for the patient's treatment should be carried out. Full advantage should be taken, if possible, of the fact that the patient's most comfortable period is usually at the completion of the ritualistic behavior.

A more serious problem that does arise at times is fatigue that occurs when the patient's behavior is so elaborate and involved that it exhausts him. A plan to guarantee the patient adequate rest should be worked out and rigidly carried through.

Physical needs. The majority of physical needs of ritualistic patients arise as a result of the compulsive act and may, therefore, be quite varied in nature. The maintenance of adequate food and fluid intake may become a problem, and if it does, feeding should be carried out on a rigid schedule. Compulsive washing may lead to problems in skin care. Compulsive picking at the body may lead to infection.

Protection. Patients in this group have two major protective needs; they must be protected from the consequences of their behavior and from the development of panic. The former, of course, will depend upon the form the compulsive behavior takes. If the patient steals compulsively, for example, no issue should be made concerning the act itself. Rather, careful observation of what is stolen and quiet return of stolen articles would be a wiser procedure. Periodic tactful search for the patient's compulsive acquisitions may be instituted. The principle involved is the avoidance of punitive measures for behavior the patient cannot control.

The avoidance of panic rests upon keeping anxiety at the lowest possible level in the patient. The particular danger point is the compulsive act itself, which should not be blocked or used in any manner to create further anxiety in the patient. The careful avoidance of contribution to the patient's sense of guilt is also important.

Group relations. The ritualistic patient tries to isolate himself from group contacts, and this tendency is to be tactfully combatted at every turn. It can be helpful to adjust routine to permit the compulsive act when and where it does not make the patient conspicuous in the eyes of the group and where and when it does not interfere with group activities. As a rule, a definite effort on the part of personnel to introduce and encourage group activities by the patient is necessary. He also needs support in group activities in which his sense of adequacy is threatened; therefore, it is sound procedure to start him with an activity in which he is already interested and has some skill. A tendency on the part of the patient to do menial tasks for other patients (self-punishment) should be calmly permitted. Unless the compulsive act itself is a sharp handicap, the patient is usually fairly well accepted by the group unless there happens to be too many members like himself. He can often be a fairly constructive group member.

Convalescence. The major emphasis during the patient's convalescence is upon satisfactory socialization with others. The patient's tendency to be impatient and to demand much of himself should be recognized, and the necessary support and encouragement should be given. He may often show contempt for the symptom he is losing and may be sharply critical of himself for having been ill. Under no circumstances should personnel agree with any such expression, but should encourage the patient with the real improvement he has shown.

Any compulsive or ritualistic behavior should be tactfully observed and reported and completely ignored as far as the patient is concerned.

References

Cameron, Norman: The psychology of behavior disorders, Boston, 1947, Houghton Mifflin Co., pp. 278-317.

Friedman, Paul: The phobias. In Arieti, Silvana, editor: American handbook of psychiatry, New York, 1959, Basic Books, Inc., vol. 1, pp. 293-306.

Noyes, Arthur P., and Kolb, Lawrence C.: Modern clinical psychiatry, ed. 6, Philadelphia, 1963, W. B. Saunders Co., pp. 443-448.

Schwartz, Morris S., and Shockley, Emmy Lanning: The nurse and the mental patient, New York, 1956, Russell Sage Foundation, pp. 182-198.

Sullivan, Harry Stack: Conceptions of modern psychiatry, Washington, D. C., 1947, William Alanson White Psychiatric Foundation, pp. 55-58.

Chapter XV

Nursing care of patients with socially aggressive patterns

Among the most fascinating and the least understood of the personality disorders is a variegated pattern of behavior dubiously called the sociopathic personality behavior disorders. If there are central characteristics for this disorder, they could probably be listed as fluent verbal behavior combined with superficial emotional responses, failure to profit from experience, antisocial behavior, and fleeting emotional involvements with other people and with social institutions. Such a combination results in seemingly inexplicable and almost self-destructive behavior in a person who sounds like any ordinary human being when you talk to him. Sociopaths are the despair of friends and relatives, psychiatrists and policemen, and the general public. The questions, What are they? Why are they the way they are? and What can be done about them? are baffling beyond description. Such limited explanations as are available at the present will be presented briefly, and the emptiness of the solution of what to do will indicate how inadequate is the current understanding of what and why.

Dynamics of development

Much of the behavior of patients whose difficulty seems to lie primarily in the area of disregard for social standards with the payment of little personal discomfort seems explicable in terms of a deep lack of emotional capacity which is not always obvious to the casual observer. The individual who does not feel so deeply as others or is unable to feel with others misses most of the important significance of human experience. Experience has not the same meaning for such a person, nor can he appreciate what is important to others. An outlook on life that does not include the usual depth of the experiences of love, hate, shame, etc., makes the integration of experience difficult and hampers incredibly the growth toward a mature personality. After all, the first steps toward growth come through strong emotional response to reward and punishment. Without the emotional component, approval and disapproval are not sufficiently strong to mold the growing individual into accepted patterns of behavior. Characteristically, patients with this defect usually show a long history of maladjustment which grows increasingly evident as they age and more mature criteria are used as a standard for comparison with their behavior. Also in keeping with this basic assumption, that the central defect in the personality structure is a severe limitation of emotional capacity, is the fact that such patients are rarely modified by experience or treatment. The need for approval as a means of security is an important motivating factor in the direction toward mental health, and such patients are not susceptible to motivation of this sort.

What causes the constriction of emotional capacity? The answer is not clear although several possible explanations hold some fruitful promise for exploration. Extremely severe emotional trauma early in life, especially in an extremely sensitive child, might possibly lead to a rejection of the emotion aspect of existence although a repression so deep and so complete of what ordinarily constitutes a major portion of experience would require very severe trauma. It is not impossible, however.

Another possibility is the effect of parents who mechanize human relationships—who are capable of living only with the intellect. The absence of warmth in parents, especially if the child is isolated from other contacts before school age, may result in personality growth being forever stunted by the effect of growing up in an emotional refrigerator. The traits of such parents are exaggerated in the child. It would be necessary, of course, for both parents to participate in such a pattern or for the pattern to be determined by one parent who completely dominated the child.

The hypothesis that patients with socially aggressive disorders are victims of some lack at birth has been advanced frequently. The theory has never been adequately proved or disproved.

As may be gathered, why a sociopath is a sociopath is a matter for investigation, rather than for discussion. We simply do not know.

Types of behavior

The types of behavior shown by patients with this particular group of disorders are not easy to describe either. There is not complete agreement on what is included in the grouping, and the types of classification within the species vary with the clinician's personal experience and attitude toward patients as well as numerous other factors. The descriptions that follow are not intended to be wholly inclusive or exclusive. A patient need not show all of them to be a sociopath, nor would the existence of other symptoms than those mentiioned exclude him from consideration as a sociopath.

Patients in this category usually possess superficial charm and good intelligence. They sound quite interesting and interested, can discuss numerous subjects, nearly always say the right thing, and say it well. That they do not mean what they say is not apparent on first or casual acquaintance. Met only on a verbal level, they seem to be thoroughly competent.

If they could live life as well as they talk it, all would be in order. These persons, however, are completely unreliable. They lack a sense of responsibility in both trivial and serious matters and further confuse observers with spasmodic periods of conforming behavior. Closer observation usually reveals that periods of conforming behavior cost the conformer little in terms of energy and nothing in terms of personal sacrifice.

A pattern of frequent failure is characteristic. Although the patient gives evidence of having the potential to succeed in his chosen field, he rarely stays with it and frequently quits for seemingly trivial causes. He lacks perseverance. He may look good for a little while, but given time, he shows his inadequacy.

Insincerity and untruthfulness are hall marks of this group of patients, Yet they sound as though they mean every word they say. It is only when they fail to carry through into behavior that the insincerity and lack of honesty become apparent. They may protest a deep affection for a spouse, spend the night with someone else, come back the next day with the same protestation of deep affection, and see no incongruity in their words and their actions. Further, they will be annoyed and righteously indignant if criticized.

A complete egocentricity is also characteristic of the sociopath. What emotional capacity he has is centered on himself, and he seems incapable of any real emotional investment in others. Deep and lasting affection for another is utterly foreign to his nature. His readiness of expression is often confused with strength of feeling. In all situations he suffers from lack of enduring emotional responses. Remorse and shame are beyond him; although he can and does convincingly apologize, he repeats his offense at the first opportunity. He learns little from experience and seems never to think of the consequences of his behavior. His antisocial acts seem often to have little reason behind them, and he shows no compunction for the pain he causes others. He usually shows impatience at the idea that he should be punished or constrained from following his wishes. His judgment is poor, and he steals when he is sure to be caught, spends his money on pleasure when he needs it to pay his bills, and repeats the same mistakes again and again. Kindness, special consideration, and trust are taken for granted and arouse no response of appreciation. His sex life is impersonal and poorly integrated. As would be suspected, he is often sexually promiscuous, but the act itself is without any deep personal significance for him. He cannot evaluate himself or his behavior realistically and rationalizes easily by way of explanation. He is irresponsible and completely undisturbed about it. He has no life plan and cannot follow one consistently. In other words, only the present is significant, the past matters little, and the future does not count.

The specific expressions of the disorder are to be found in sexual promiscuity and perversions, in unnecessary lying, in stealing, in recklessness that seems foolish and without reason, and in the indiscriminate use of drugs and alcohol. It is seen in a whole range of minor and major infractions of the law, such as forgeries, arson, assault, and robbery. It is seen in the constant use of other people for personal and casual satisfaction.

By way of summary, behavior characterized by the following traits, shown in social aggression rather than psychotic symptoms, is considered sociopathic: inability to profit from experience, poor judgment, living for the present, emotional deficiency with cold-blooded self-centeredness and little or no capacity for remorse, quick and facile emotional responses without depth or duration, amorality, lack of a sense of responsibility, explosiveness under pressure, and a tendency to repeat mistakes. Many of these characteristics are not obvious on first acquaintance, and it is only when the patient is better known that his difficulties become obvious.

Problems of therapy

The inadequate knowledge concerning the so-called sociopathic personalities may be one of the reasons for the generally held nihilistic attitude toward therapy. Few of these patients are ever completely cured. The sociopath's uncooperativness toward treatment and his peculiar legal status make it exceedingly difficult to get him under treatment and to keep him there.

Phychiatrists do not agree on much of anything except that the treatment of sociopaths is a difficult task. In fact, some of them go so far as to say that, if a sociopath recovers and makes a good social adjustment, the diagnosis was wrong. In recent years a somewhat more hopeful attitude has been expressed from several quarters, but such voices are few. This attitude is understandable in view of the fact that so little is known concerning causative factors in the development of a sociopathic personality. When our state of knowledge expands, as it has recently in so many other areas of personality disorders, there may occur a marked advance in the therapy of patients with aggressive personality disorders.

The legal status of the sociopath has been a factor in limiting the amount of study and research devoted to his problems. Such patients are not, by legal definition, psychotic, which makes them ineligible for psychiatric hospitalization except in private institutions where the cost of care is prohibitive. The great majority of psychiatric patients are in governmental hospitals of one type or another, where sociopaths cannot remain unless their problems are complicated by a psychotic episode. Under such circumstances relatively little effort has been expended on the problem of understanding the sociopath since more extensive and urgent problems of other types of disorders confront the psychiatric health team in their working environment.

Because of their inability to abide by rules and regulations which conflict with their impulses and immediate wishes, sociopaths frequently come into conflict with the law, which results in jail sentences. It is also true that many of these patients show real ability at evading paying the consequences of their behavior. Although they *do* serve jail sentences, there are many more occasions in which additional or longer penalties would have seemed indicated.

Even though the personal history may indicate quite clearly that society needs protection from the sociopathic person and will continue to need protection during his lifetime, the patient can be sentenced only for the period his particular offense merits and then must be released, to transgress again. This is not to imply that all sociopaths are criminals, nor that all criminals are sociopaths. However, many of them do come in conflict with the law and pose a severe problem in rehabilitation.

Thus there is no place where adequate measures can be taken to force the sociopath under long-range treatment and keep him there. And, if all treatment fails, there is no way to adequately protect the patient from himself and society from him. Therapy is frustrated by the patient's inability to integrate new experience and alter his personality development through corrective experience. He does not profit by mistakes, and thus his poor judgment has little opportunity to improve. The traits that characterize his developmental defect operate to prevent his improvement.

Nursing care

In view of the preceding, it must be understood that what is said here concerning the nursing care of sociopathic patients is a series of tentative suggestions that may prove false in any specific instance. What is suggested should be checked carefully against experience and revised as necessary.

Actually, relatively few sociopaths will be found in psychiatric hospitals. Because their incidence in the general population is not small, it is important to recognize them for what they are and to be able to identify them. They make poor friends, poor wives and husbands, and the payment for becoming emotionally involved with them comes high in personal unhappiness.

Psychotherapeutic environment. In our present state of knowledge, about all we can say concerning the type of environment necessary for a sociopathic personality is that it should provide a considerable degree of control over the patient. In line with developing knowledge, however, it seems safe to add that the environment should also be one in which the atmosphere is oriented toward understanding of the fact that the patient's behavior is symptomatic of a personality defect and in which careful observation and study of the patient is possible.

It is not known whether the cultural milieu of a psychiatric hospital which abounds with frankly psychotic patients is the best place for attempted treatment of sociopathic personalities. It may be that a different type of institution needs to be developed.

Interpersonal relationships. The major problem in interpersonal relationships with sociopathic personalities is to avoid being taken in by their smooth and often charming exteriors. With their verbal fluency and seemingly intact intelligence, they often appear and look extremely well adjusted and give the impression of being very nice people who have wandered into the hospital by mistake. They are quite plausible and play neatly on the sympathies of personnel. The danger in being taken in lies in the fact that the sociopath uses other people ruthlessly and without remorse for his own purposes. When a member of the staff is suddenly confronted with the patient's defects, the natural reaction is to apply normal standards of conduct for judgment and to be quite angry. If the staff expects the patient to lie, steal, to stir up trouble, and to project his defects to personnel, it is much easier to accept the patient's behavior quietly and not put any additional pressure on him. The sociopath tends to be explosive under pressure.

It should also be kept in mind that the sociopath's feeling about rules and regulations is that they exist to be broken. While seeming to conform, they manage to evade many requirements and reveal their success as a rule where it can be most embarrassing to the victim they outwitted. A resentment of authority and any form of restraint should be expected and quietly accepted. The more intelligent form their rebellion takes makes it somewhat harder to accept than the open rebellion expressed by the psychotic patient. Going along with the patient in his neat rationalization of his objection to routine should be avoided. A certain quiet firmness should be maintained constantly with the patient.

In other words, so far as we now know, the approach to be used with the sociopathic personality is to remain constantly on guard in order to be able to quietly accept his amoral or antisocial behavior when it does appear. On the surface he seems so charmingly normal that the tendency to retaliate when he does not wear well is hard to curb. The patient needs acceptance as he is, and it is not especially good for him to have his capacities overestimated.

Physical needs. A daily routine stressing good health habits should be carried out. As a rule, the sociopath is physically healthy and able to care for his own personal needs. If physical defects or illnesses are present, every effort should be made to return the patient to a normal state of health and improve his physical status.

Protection. The protective needs of the sociopath are usually more in the nature of protecting others from him. He should be protected from the results of indulging in impulsive expression of primitive tendencies. It should be remembered that most of the difficulty for such patients is in the area of adjusting to social control applied to themselves or others.

The sociopath is often casually cruel to others, and sensitive patients may need to be protected from contact with him. He is often the source of forbidden materials for such patients, and this trait should be carefully watched for and guarded against. He is the person who finds razor blades for the depressed patient and matches for the confused and bewildered patient who is unsafe with them.

Group relations. The sociopath, as a rule, makes a good initial impression on the group, but he does not wear well. He often causes arguments without being involved himself, he helps other patients break rules and laughs at their resulting difficulties, and he makes fun of the psychotic ideas of patients. He is an extremely disruptive group member and needs careful study to keep him constructively occupied without doing it at someone else's expense. His defective social judgment becomes most apparent in his group relationships. He often shows a tendency in a hospital situation to identify himself with personnel and should not be encouraged in the practice if the effect is detrimental to other patients. If it is not, however, this trait can be used to keep the patient constructively occupied.

Convalescence. Too much should not be expected of the patient during his convalescence, nor should he be trusted too far. Firmness in keeping the patient on routine will still be necessary, and every encouragement to help the patient accept continued treatment should be given him. Above all, careful and objective observation of the patient and detailed charting are important. They are badly needed resources for research in this particular area.

References

Block, Donald A.: Sex crimes and criminals, American Journal of Nursing **53**:440-442, Sept. 1953.

Cleckley, Hervey M.: Psychopathic states. In Arieti, Silvana, editor: American handbook of psychiatry, New York, 1959, Basic Books, Inc., vol. 1, pp. 567-588.

Cleckley, Hervey M.: The mask of sanity, ed. 3, St. Louis, 1955, The C. V. Mosby Co.

Lindner, Robert: Rebel without a cause, New York, 1944, Grune & Stratton, Inc.

Noyes, Arthur P., and Kolb, Lawrence C.: Modern clinical psychiatry, ed. 6, Philadelphia, 1963, W. B. Saunders Co., pp. 460-471.

Chapter XVI

Nursing care in somatic procedures

Certain somatic procedures in the treatment of functional behavior disorders have been developed; some are based on sound physiologic principles and some on clinical experience. Among these somatic procedures are some of the more dramatic forms of psychiatric therapy: electric and insulin shock, psychosurgery, and the new tranquilizing drugs. These have been developed through observation, by accident, and on questionable theory, but nonetheless are being used extensively on empirical grounds. Shock therapy and psychosurgery have contributed to the improvement of the clinical status of patients although why they have remains a moot point.

Insulin shock treatment

Insulin had previously been used in the symptomatic treatment of mental illness, especially for its sedative effect on excited patients and its stimulating effect on patients with a poor nutritional status, and in the treatment of drug addiction. Manfred Sakel, of the University Clinic of Vienna, noticed that deeper hypoglycemic effects, occurring accidentally, were apparently correlated with an improvement in the clinical status of patients. With this observation in mind, Sakel used insulin coma, until then avoided, with varying types of patients in a curative effort. His report in 1933 marked the beginning of the shock era of treatment in psychiatry. The basic method of treatment devised by Sakel is still used.

The use of insulin coma spread rapidly, and the treatment was used at one time or another on patients with practically all types of psychoses. Gradually criteria for its use were developed, and insulin shock has become a fairly respectable treatment technique. Experience has shown it to be most effective in the treatment of patients who show withdrawn patterns of behavior. The use of insulin shock therapy has decreased in recent years as a result of the effectiveness of the tranquilizing drugs, whose use is far less dangerous and less complex medically. Another factor in the decreased use is undoubtedly the great cost in personnel and time involved in insulin therapy. Insulin shock therapy, however, is still considered to be important.

Insulin shock consists of the production of a state of coma in fasting patients by the injection of a fairly large dose of insulin. The coma is terminated by the administration of sugar in a readily absorbable form, the route of administration depending upon the condition of the patient. The usual procedure is to start the patient on a small dose of insulin and build up the amount day by day until coma results. The amount of insulin required to produce coma varies markedly from patient to patient; 60 units or less of regular insulin are sufficient to cause coma for some patients, whereas other patients may need several hundred units.

The most commonly used approach to the production of coma is the rapid induction method. Patients are given small doses of insulin at the start, the dosage is doubled until 300 to 400 units are reached, and increases of 100 to 200 units daily are used until coma appears about two or three hours after injection. Coma usually occurs in seven to ten days. The patient is allowed to reach a state of coma, and the treatment is then terminated for the first time. (The most precarious stage of insulin shock therapy is during the early coma phase.) The coma periods are gradually extended to an hour, and treatment is continued until the patient has had fifty hours of coma. The average dose required to produce coma is around 200 to 400 units of insulin although the range is 10 to 20 units up to 2,000 to 4,000 units. Variations of the procedure here described appear in individual institutions.

Insulin shock treatment can only be given in a fully equipped unit within a hospital where a trained team of physicians, nurses, and attendants is available to give safe care. The procedure can be a dangerous one. Alert observation and facilities for prompt emergency treatment are musts. For this reason, the use of insulin shock was somewhat curbed during World War II due to a lack of medical and nursing personnel.

Complications occurring in the use of insulin shock therapy include hyperexcitable states that can be serious enough to cause cardiac collapse, convulsions, prolonged or irreversible coma, and after reactions. The most serious and the least common is prolonged or irreversible coma. Fortunately, as teams of doctors and nurses have learned more about insulin coma therapy, the incidence of irreversible coma has decreased. The patient fails to regain consciousness, shows signs of central nervous system involvement, cyanosis, elevated temperature, respiratory impairment, and sometimes convulsions to the extent of status epilepticus. This calls for intensive medical and nursing care. Convulsions may also occur during the period of coma, and patients not infrequently show improvement in their behavior afterward. However, convulsions can indicate difficulty, and the later in the coma the convulsion appears, the more likely it is to be a danger sign. Once it is known that the patient tends to have convulsions during coma, preventive measures can be taken by the use of Dilantin or barbiturates. Extremely hyperexcitable states with sharply increased motor activity usually call for intervention since insulin coma by itself places a heavy stress on the cardiovascular and central nervous systems. Afterreactions include tremor, weakness, excessive perspiration, drowsiness, sleepiness, or faintness that may progress to a full-fledged insulin reaction with coma. If they are noticed, such reactions are easily controlled by glucose administration. They may occur during the twenty-four hour period following treatment.

As indicated, insulin shock has proved most effective in the treatment of withdrawal patterns of behavior. However, even in this group of patients, it is most effective with those patients whose prognosis would be best regardless of the type of therapeutic approach. Although the outcome of treatment for any individual patient cannot be accurately predicted, the following conditions give the patient a good statistical opportunity for recovery: illness of one year's duration or less, good adjustment previous to illness, strong emotional response to illness, definite environmental precipitating factors, and an acute onset.

On the basis of what is known at present, insulin shock treatment is an adjunct to psychiatric therapy, and its primary function is to make the patient accessible to psychotherapy and other forms of psychiatric treatment. It hastens recovery and helps to reduce the length of hospitalization. The long range value of insulin shock therapy is not yet fully determined. The relapse rate is high, and the second course of treatment is usually not so effective as the first.

Nursing care. Orientation of the patient to the treatment is part of his nursing care since a treatment which produces unconsciousness is almost certain to have deep significance for the patient. Even though the patient may appear to have little interest in or response to an explanation, it is always given since we know definitely that some patients of this type are fully alert to their environment, and we strongly suspect that others are as well. Realistic reassurance in regard to the treatment only should be given.

The administration of insulin requires certain precautions. The medication must be given intramuscularly and deeply so. For this reason, the buttocks are the usual choice of site of administration. Care must be taken to avoid injection of insulin into fatty surface tissues. If the dose is large, a divided dose with two or more injections may be used. The patient should be observed for signs of an allergic response to insulin, usually indicated by welts at the site of the injection or the appearance of hives elsewhere on the body. In case of such a reaction, a prompt report should be made to the physician in charge. The usual procedure is for the insulin to be given to a fasting patient early in the morning on the ward and then later for the patient to be sent to the insulin treatment unit.

Upon arrival in the treatment unit, the patient should be put to bed, and hospital gowns should be used in preference to the patient's own clothing. Very close observation of the patient's condition should be maintained. Depending upon the institution, the patient may or may not be restrained for the treatment. The particular signs accepted by the physician as an indication of coma should be reported and recorded as they occur. Generally accepted signs of coma are loss of the pain reflex on eyeball pressure, loss of light accommodation in the eye, failure to react to a sharp flick of the fingernail on the cheek, and failure to respond to a sharp noise near the ear. During coma the patient should be kept in bed with the head slightly elevated and turned to one side to prevent aspiration of mucus. Suction should be used to clear the throat if necessary. Throughout the treatment the patient should be adequately covered with blankets and protected from drafts since perspiration is profuse, and the susceptibility to chills is marked. Convulsions may occur and are usually heralded by tonic spasms. A mouth gag should be inserted and held in place, and if possible, the extremities should be controlled to prevent dislocation or fractures. A convulsion is sometimes an indication for termination.

The nurse should be prepared to assist with termination of the coma. In the early stages of treatment the patient may be able to drink a sugar solution. If coma is present, nasal gavage is ordinarily used, and in emergencies intravenous glucose is given. In any case, it is the responsibility of the nurse to have everything prepared for emergency measures if they should be necessary. If a patient does not react in fifteen to twenty minutes following nasal gavage, the physician should be notified since the administration of intravenous glucose is indicated in such instances.

After termination of the coma, the patient should be wrapped in warm dry blankets and fed a substantial meal. If he is nauseated, feeding should not be forced to the point of vomiting since nothing constructive would be accomplished. However, more intake is needed than that given in the termination of the coma since the sugar given by that method is rapidly absorbed and used, and the patient needs a further cushion, more slowly absorbed, for the period when the glucose or dextrose given earlier has been used. The patient's behavior following termination should be carefully noted and charted.

After a meal patients should be showered and dressed, and then a program of activities to exploit their greater accessibility should be instituted. Patients should have between-meal nourishment and should be watched at all times for delayed shock reactions.

It is important to learn the patient's usual course during insulin shock treatment since the pattern tends to remain the same for each patient. Any deviation from the usual, no matter how slight, should be reported.

Insulin subshock treatment

Several types of insulin treatment short of shock therapy are being used, although their use, too, is decreasing. The amount of insulin given is comparatively small and is calculated to produce hypoglycemia without permitting the patient to go into coma. The treatment is not a substitute for insulin shock therapy but is used for its sedative effect in the reduction of anxiety and overactivity. Subshock or subcoma treatment is used primarily as a supportive measure, and its ultimate purpose is to make the patient accessible to psychotherapy.

There are numerous variations of the treatment, including ambulatory insulin treatment in which the patient is permitted to be up and about and engage in his usual activities until the hypoglycemic reaction appears. In subcoma treatment, the patient usually remains in bed until the reaction is terminated. The stage at which termination is ordered depends upon the physician and the institution. Some physicians prefer to terminate after one-half hour of the reaction and others on the basis of symptoms presented. Some prefer that termination occur well in advance of the possibility of coma, and others like to let the patient get to the very edge of coma before termination of treatment. In addition to the physician's preference, the condition of the patient may be a factor in deciding such issues.

Subshock or ambulatory insulin treatment is ordinarily a daily procedure. The length of treatment varies according to the experience of the staff and the condition of the patient. In chronic illness, the treatment may continue for a year or more when the purpose is to help the patient control himself. A frank therapeutic course may be given in several months or may consist of one hundred or more injections. The individual treatment period usually lasts from two and one-half to three and one-half hours. The time of administration and termination will depend largely upon the staff of the institution. If the night staff is adequate, the treatment may start early so that the patient is able to eat his breakfast at the regular hour. Otherwise, the treatment will begin when the day staff reports on duty, and breakfast will be served at midmorning. The termination is accomplished by the patient's drinking a glucose solution, usually 1 gm. of glucose per unit of insulin. Gavages and intravenous glucose should always be available in case of emergencies, which do occur.

Nursing care. Orientation to the procedure to help the patient know what to expect is essential since the symptoms of hypoglycemia may frighten him when they do occur, especially if he does not know what they are. Careful observation of the patient is necessary, of course, and should be especially intense after the first signs of the reaction appear. Each patient, as a rule, has his own pattern of response, and the nurse should be thoroughly familiar with it. Any unusual variation should be promptly reported. The expected symptoms are weakness, increased perspiration, hunger, restlessness, tremors, twitching, thickening speech, and drowsiness.

The patient's behavior should be charted in detail during the treatment. After treatment, the patient should be encouraged to participate in activities and should be observed for any signs of a secondary hypoglycemic reaction. If any symptoms do occur, glucose should be given orally promptly.

Electroshock therapy

Based on the inaccurate conclusion that epilepsy, a convulsive disorder, was antagonistic to certain types of mental illness, an attempt to treat withdrawal patterns of behavior disorders with artificially induced convulsions was undertaken. Von Meduna reported in 1935 on the use of camphor and Metrazol to produce convulsions as a method of treatment. One of the disadvantages of the use of these drugs was a feeling of impending doom that the patient experienced between the injection and the time the convulsion actually started. In 1937 Cerletti and Bini suggested the use of an electric current as the convulsive stimuli, and electroshock therapy rapidly replaced the use of drugs. Experience has shown it to be most effective in the treatment of both agitated and retarded depressions and to a lesser degree in the treatment of overactivity.

The procedure itself consists of the production of a typical grand mal convulsion by the application of an electric current through electrodes placed on the patient's temples. The convulsive threshold varies from patient to patient; therefore the amount of current required varies from patient to patient. The convulsion itself starts with a tonic spasm of the entire body and is followed by a series of clonic, jerking motions most marked in the extremities. The patient remains unconscious for several minutes following treatment and is usually quite confused as he recovers. He is able to be up and about in approximately thirty minutes although he may need assistance at first.

The course of treatment again varies, being from six to twenty shocks. Some physicians may go well beyond twenty shocks for an individual patient, and the patient may also receive more than one course of treatment. It is customary to give three treatments a week. Electroshock may also be given on a maintenance basis both in the hospital and in the outpatient department although its use for this purpose is decreasing. In such instances, the patient may receive a single treatment at regular intervals, such as every two weeks, every month, or every other month. In marked overactivity that may constitute a real danger to the patient, treatments may be given on successive days or several treatments on one day until the overactivity subsides below the danger point.

The use of muscle relaxant drugs to reduce the possibilities of fracture and the severity of muscle contractions in electroconvulsive therapy has been explored. One of the first drugs used was curare, most often in the form of Intocostrin. Since curare itself is a rather dangerous drug with the potential complication of respiratory paralysis, it has largely been replaced by succinylcholine (Anectine) used in conjunction with Pentothal Sodium. Some psychiatrists use muscle relaxant drugs routinely, whereas others feel the use of the drugs complicates the treatment through added potential danger. Many prefer no premedications and use them only when there is some specific indication.

The commonest complication in the use of electroshock therapy is compression fracture of the spine in the middorsal region, usually between the fourth and eighth thoracic vertebrae. Such fractures are most frequently asymptomatic and of little clinical significance. Rarely, but more serious, fractures of the humerus or femur occur. Actually, electroshock therapy is a fairly safe procedure, and many conditions once considered contraindications for its use have been removed from the list. Among the few conditions still considered contraindications are recent coronary thrombosis, cardiac decompensation, and unhealed bone fractures.

Electroshock therapy may also be used in combination with insulin shock. Two methods are used. The electroshock treatment may be used on one day and insulin the next day, or the electroshock may be given just before terminating the insulin coma. The combined use was developed in the therapy of patients who tended to relapse.

Nursing care. Patients receiving electroshock therapy need a great deal of reassurance because of the marked memory defect that accompanies the treatment and because of the general tendency of persons to fear the loss of consciousness. There is usually some apprehension in regard to the convulsion as well since most patients know that a convulsion will occur.

The preparation for the treatment is both physical and psychologic. Breakfast should either be very light or completely withheld. All dentures should be removed, and nothing loose should be in the patient's mouth during the convulsion. All metal objects, such as bobby pins and clips, should be removed from the patient's hair. Clothing should be loose. The commonest psychologic problem is the patient's apprehension in regard to the treatment. Pleasant surroundings in which to await treatment and agreeable diversion to keep the patient occupied should be provided.

Nursing care during the actual convulsion consists of control of the patient's body to prevent fractures or other injuries. The shoulders should be gently held in place and the pelvis loosely so. During the clonic phase of the convulsion, the arms and legs should be permitted rather free motion, but should be guided to prevent adduction from the body plane if possible. Tight restriction of the body movements during the convulsion may contribute to fractures. A mouth gag, preferably of soft rubber covered with gauze, is kept inserted between the teeth during treatment. If the patient refuses to bite down on the gag before the treatment is started, it is usually possible to insert the gag during the tonic phase of the convulsion when the patient shows the characteristic tonic yawn. Upward pressure should be applied to the chin to prevent dislocation of the jaw or tongue swallowing. As soon as the convulsion ends, the patient's head should be turned on one side since breathing is stertorous, and mucus tends to collect in the back of the throat.

The patient should be closely observed following the convulsion in order to prevent injury and to give reassurance as needed. Some patients are extremely restless and overactive and can injure themselves seriously while thrashing about. The pattern of behavior postconvulsively is usually typical for each patient so that it is fairly easy to know which patients need the closest observation. When the patient is able to answer simple questions, he can usually be helped out of the treatment room.

The patient is then returned to his unit, where he is showered, dressed, and fed. Because of his confusion and memory defect, he will probably need reassurance. The regular program of activities should be followed for the rest of the day. During the course of treatment the patient is likely to become more accessible so that this period should be thoroughly exploited to establish good relationships and to give the patient a sense of being with interested and understanding company.

Psychosurgery

A surgical approach to the treatment of mental illness was begun by Egas Moniz, a Portuguese psychiatrist, who reported the use of prefrontal lobotomy in 1935. The next year the procedure was introduced in the United States by Freeman and Watts. The use of psychosurgery has decreased with the advent of the tranquilizing drugs.

In prefrontal lobotomy, the association fibers between the frontal lobes and the thalamus are severed. Although the specific functions of the frontal lobes are not clearly understood, there is general agreement that the thalamus is the place where emotional responses are invested in ideas and sensations. The surgical procedure is thus an effort to detach the emotional component of the psychosis and enable the patient to live more comfortably. The operation is performed through burr holes in the skull, and the association fibers are cut in the plane of the coronal suture.

Other surgical procedures, based on the same principle, have been developed. Topectomy consists of the removal of areas of cortex in the frontal lobes. In thalamotomy, an electric needle is inserted in the thalamus to destroy some of the tissue and thus reduce the patient's emotional tension. Transorbital lobotomy consists of severing the association fibers from above the eye. This procedure, introduced by Freeman and Watts, is probably more extensively used than any other.

Patients who retain a strong emotional reaction to their illness and to their psychotic ideas have responded best to psychosurgery. Patients with agitated depressions, withdrawal, and projective patterns have tended to show improvement. However, it must be kept in mind that, while psychosurgery may result in the patient's being able to return to the community, he is very likely to show some deterioration from his prepsychotic level of behavior as a result of the operation. Unpleasant traits are likely to be magnified, social inhibitions may be somewhat lessened, and the ability to carry out complex tasks may be reduced. Nevertheless, when all other forms of treatment have been tried and have failed, and the patient is markedly uncomfortable in his illness, psychosurgery offers a hope of some improvement.

Nursing care. The immediate postoperative nursing care of patients with a prefrontal lobotomy is surgical in nature. Temperature, pulse, respiration, and blood pressure are checked at frequent intervals. Danger signs are pulse rate below 60 or above 120, temperature over 102° F., sudden drop in blood pressure or a rise in systolic pressure over 150, continued vomiting, failure to regain consciousness in three or four hours, and after the return to consciousness marked restlessness followed by drowsiness or unconsciousness. After reacting, the patient is likely to be confused and disoriented and needs reassurance and tactful encouragement to refrain from pulling at his bandage or removing it. Ordinarily the patient is allowed out of bed briefly the day of operation or the first postoperative day, and every effort is made to get the patient ambulatory as soon as possible. While the patient does remain in bed, crayons and drawing paper, bright objects, rag dolls or teddy bears, building blocks, or similar articles are used to keep him occupied, to keep his bandage intact, and to combat masturbatory activity.

Following the operation most patients are regressed, some to a greater degree than others. The major task in nursing care is resocialization through habit training. Incontinence, exceedingly common, gradually comes under control through regular toilet periods. Feeding habits are poor, and training in table manners is necessary. The biggest difficulty in the habit-training program is encountered in the patient's inertia, procrastination, and complete lack of regard for time. It becomes necessary to initiate activity for the patient and to help him carry through. Negativism also frequently presents a problem and must be met firmly. The convalescent period for a patient who has undergone a prefrontal lobotomy is a period of growing up again, a period of reacquiring all the basic social skills. It is quite important during this period that the patient have a planned schedule of activities and adequate supervision designed to encourage his assumption of responsibility for his own activities.

Narcoanalysis

The use of various drugs in the treatment of mental illness dates as far back as the history of psychiatry. One particular use of barbiturates—the intravenous injection of Sodium Amytal and Pentothal Sodium—received a tremendous impetus during World War II and resulted in making the procedure known as narcoanalysis a respectable and effective adjunct to psychiatric therapy. In addition to the use of barbiturates as simple narcotics and anticonvulsants, the two previously mentioned drugs in this category are now used in establishing contact with suspicious and inaccessible patients, in shortening therapy by overcoming resistance, and as a first-aid measure in traumatic situations such as combat experience in war. The barbiturates are central nervous system depressants and have some effects that are comparable to hypnosis. Patients' inhibitions are often lessened, and they are able to discuss material that they cannot otherwise. They may also be able to recall experiences that have been repressed, and they may become suggestible and accept reassurance and constructive interpretation of what has happened to them.

Narcoanalysis consists of the intravenous injection of Sodium Amytal or Pentothal Sodium, given very slowly. The dose required to produce results varies widely, and the amount given is determined by the degree of relaxation and accessibility of the patient. The needle remains inserted in the vein during the treatment so that further medication may be given to maintain the patient at the desired level. The physician then directs questions or conversation to sensitive areas, either to elicit desired information for his own use in planning therapy or to permit the patient to recall painful experiences. Reassurance and suggested synthesis of the experience for a more constructive attitude on the part of the patient are given before the treatment ends. A very definite attempt to establish rapport with the patient is integrated into the procedure. The treatment may be used only once or a few times with a patient, or a series of injections may be given.

Nursing care. In narcoanalysis, the nurse should be alert to the opportunity to establish rapport with the patient. She should also recognize the patient's greater suggestibility and be careful to maintain a positive and reassuring attitude. Indecision and doubt on her part immediately following the treatment may help to unsettle the patient somewhat. Particular care should also be taken in regard to material discussed by the patient if the nurse should be aware of it. The choice of bringing up such topics should be left to the patient and not referred to unless the patient himself mentions it.

Psychopharmacology

The new developments in psychopharmacology, with their dramatic effect on the behavior of psychotic patients, have stirred the hopes of many patients and families.

The tranquilizers, or ataraxics, are sedative agents that reduce anxiety, agitation, and overactivity. Ataraxia, which is Greek in origin, denotes calm, peace of mind, and lack of confusion. The energizers or euphoriants are compounds that have an opposite effect. They are stimulants which aid in alleviating depression and fatigue.

Two major limitations concerning these drugs must be kept in mind. First, it is too early to evaluate the long-range effectiveness of these agents. Second, these drugs are not cures for mental illness, regardless of their "miracle" effect. How these diverse agents produce the results that they do is only partly known, and in some cases, their effect has been ascertained by clinical observation, rather than by conclusive experimental data.

The ataractic drugs. As so frequently happens, the beginning use of the tranquilizing drugs in the field of psychiatry came about by accident. They were known and used in general medicine before their value to psychiatry was discovered.

For many centuries in India, snakeroot, a native shrub, has been known for its healing powers in conditions of the mind and body. *Rauwolfia ser-*

pentina was first described by Dr. Leonard Rauwolf in 1582. In 1931, Gananath Sen and Kartick Chandra Bose demonstrated the effectiveness of one of the alkaloids from *Rauwolfia serpentina* in reducing hypertension. The tranquilizing side effect of the drug was noted, and its application to psychiatric therapy was investigated. In 1952, a group of scientists working in Switzerland extracted reserpine from the snakeroot plant. In 1953, the use of reserpine was begun in the United States by Nathan Kline. Reserpine may be considered typical of the numerous Rauwolfia alkaloids and is known by the trade name of Serpasil. Reserpine, which acts on the central nervous system and the peripheral autonomic nervous system, produces the following effects: reduced blood pressure, slower heart rate, lowered body temperature, increased gastrointestinal activity, constricted pupils, lowered convulsive threshold, reduced psychomotor activity, reduced tension, and reduced aggressiveness and hostility. It may be administered orally or intramuscularly. The effects of this drug are observed in calm, relaxed behavior, a general sense of well-being, and relief from anxiety and agitation. It has a mild sedative effect which permits the patient to remain alert without clouding the consciousness. The dosage administered is usually determined by the symptoms and the patient's response to the medication. When massive doses are given, three phases have been observed.

1. *Sedative phase.* This phase appears immediately or after several days, produces drowsiness, and reduces agitation and overactivity.
2. *Turbulent phase.* This phase may last from several hours to several weeks. The patient appears to become worse. He complains of tremors, dizziness, restlessness, and an increase in delusions and hallucinations. Impulsive outbursts may occur. Despite this phase, the drug is not reduced unless physical symptoms appear.
3. *Integrative phase.* In this phase, the turbulent phase slowly subsides, and the patient improves. The hallucinations and delusions seem less manifest, and the patient again becomes calm, amenable, and accessible. Most patients continue on a maintenance dose of reserpine.

These phases are not the usual course for all patients. Each patient responds in his own way; whereas one patient may remain in the first phase and another in the second, neither one may attain the integrative phase. Such a response may indicate the use of other tranquilizers. However, if other drugs have been used without improvement, the patient may be maintained on a dose of reserpine which keeps him in the sedative phase.

There are many side effects associated with this drug which preclude it as an ideal agent. Nasal stuffiness, nose bleeds, and dryness of the mouth are some of the distressing symptoms. The hypotensive action of this drug may create problems for certain patients. Regular blood pressure checkups should be made. Gastic irritation, nausea, vomiting, diarrhea, and constipation are some gastrointestinal disturbances which require investigation with regard to the patient's over-all condition. Parkinsonism may also develop as a complication. In addition, it is important to note that reserpine may cause a depressive reaction rather than the hoped for well-being. Careful observation should be given to any signs of melancholia, fear, or expression of futility. Suicidal precautions should be taken. For this reason reserpine is seldom given to a depressed patient.

A second category of tranquilizers is the phenothiazines. Chlorpromazine hydrochloride (Thorazine) was discovered during an investigation of their antihistaminic action by a group of French scientists. This drug was first used in surgery, where the tranquilizing. effect was noted. Two French psychiatrists, Delay and Deniker, began using chlorpromazine alone for agitated geriatric patients, and the favorable reports of their work stimulated widespread research with the drug.

Thorazine, a central nervous system depressant, produces sedation and like reserpine does not cloud consciousness. It is particularly helpful in the treatment of acute anxiety, panic, tension, and overactivity because it takes hold almost immediately. The relaxing, calming effect has been advantageous in the treatment of manic, schizophrenic, and agitated patients. This drug has been the cause of depression in some patients, and for this reason it is avoided when depressed elements are known or observable. This effect should be watched for by nursing personnel since suicide may be the consequence.

The use of Thorázine concomittantly with other medications has proved an aid in general medicine. Administered with narcotics, it assists in relieving pain and requires a smaller dose of narcotics. It has also been used as an aid in a more comfortable, less fearful experience during childbirth. Thorazine may be administered orally or intramuscularly. An intramuscular dose should be injected slowly, and the site should be massaged slowly on completion of the injection. Should there be irritation at the site, a more dilute solution (with saline) may be considered, and the physician should be consulted. Caution should be taken to store chlorpromazine in a dark place since it decomposes rather readily. The nurse should always check and dispose of any vials which may be discolored. As with reserpine, the dosage is highly variable and is usually determined by the clinical response.

This compound, more than reserpine, has many and sometimes dangerous side effects. Blood dyscrasias, jaundice of the retention type, orthostatic hypotension, Parkinsonism, dermatitis, photosensitivity, and tachycardia are some of the known complications. Drowsinss, nausea, vomiting, tremors, edema, and polyuria are some of the temporary complaints which may accompany the administration of large doses. Nurses are cautioned to handle this medication with care and to avoid the possibility of contact dermatitis. Again it must be stressed that nurses and other personnel must be alert and attentive to both physical and behavioral changes which may occur in patients on tranquilizing drugs.

The propanediols are a third category of the ataraxics. Meprobamate

(Miltown and Equanil) is an ester of the propanediol dicarbamate compound related to mephenesin. Its ability to cause muscular relaxation makes this agent a valuable drug in the treatment of anxiety and tension states. It is widely used in the treatment of tension headaches due to muscular contraction, low back pain due to muscle tension, pylorospasm, recurrent blushing, and a variety of other conditions due to muscular tension.

The side effects are mainly drowsiness and weakness at the onset of therapy and an occasional bout of gastric distress. Allergic skin reactions have been reported to occur.

The diphenylmethan derivatives, which include azacyclonol (Frenquel), benactyzine (Suavitil), and hydroxyzine (Atarax), are a somewhat newer category of tranquilizers. Frenquel has been found to relieve acute confusional states and for this reason has been used primarily in the treatment of schizophrenic disorders, occasionally for patients with delirium tremens, and for some senile patients who are experiencing confusion.

In 1936 Suavitil was used as an atropine-like local anesthetic drug. It has the ability to reduce tension and is frequently used in combination with other sedatives or hypnotics.

Atarax is another mild tranquilizer and has been used in combination with *Rauwolfia serpentina*.

These last three drugs have few if any side effects. Drowsiness is occasionally observed. Reports and findings on these three compounds are even less conclusive than those previously discussed.

Although the tranquilizers have made a great contribution to the control of agitation, anxiety, and tension, their side effects have caused numerous cases of depression. It is this problem which has prompted investigations into euphoriant or energizing agents. The amphetamine series of drugs are known and are helpful; however, they contribute many undesirable side effects. Some of the newer stimulating drugs which alleviate feelings of depression and fatigue are Ritalin and Meratran.

They have been used in the treatment of depressions with very satisfactory results and have been of great value in alleviating the depression, drowsiness, and fatigue induced by Thorazine and reserpine. Both have a low toxicity and unpleasant side reactions, such as tension, restlessness, and emotional lability, have been infrequent in occurrence. These drugs are contraindicated for patients who are tense, anxious, and agitated since these drugs may increase their symptoms.

Dosage, as with the tranquilizers, is an individual matter based on the reaction of the patient, the reporting of personnel, and the judgment of the physician.

In the complexity and newness of psychopharmacology, a few important principles should be kept in mind with reference to use.

1. Improvement is usually related to the alleviation of observable behavioral symptoms and not to the removal of the cause of illness.

2. Dosage is dependent on the therapeutic response of the patient. Changes are made for each individual patient.
3. The sedative effect permits easy awakening and does not cloud consciousness.
4. Unpleasant side reactions do occur but may disappear with continued treatment. If they persist, the drug should be stopped.
5. Habituation seldom occurs.
6. Fatalities have been very rare; consequently the use of these drugs is considered relatively safe.
7. As an adjunct in psychotherapy, these agents can greatly improve the patients' prognosis.

Nursing care. The widespread use of these drugs as a valuable adjunct to psychotherapy involves serious consideration for the nurse. Since these drugs produce such a dramatic change in the behavior of most patients, the nurse should engage in some deep introspection. As a person and a nurse, how does she feel about these agents in the treatment of patients? Does she have adequate knowledge about the drugs—their administration, action, characteristics, and complications? What greater opportunities does she have to utilize the principles of psychiatric nursing with patients now who were inaccessible because of the nature of their symptoms?

It is a known fact that the attitude of the nurse administering a medication could produce minimal or maximal results from the drug. The common practice of administering medications *en masse,* as done in many hosiptals, could sabotage maximal effectiveness. Their major contribution is to produce within the patient the ability to participate in his environment and so begin to help himself. What better opportunity could the nurse find to encourage the patient toward this end?

Care and caution should be taken in the administration of these drugs. Dosage continues to be an individual matter for the most part. Physicians base their orders on the effect of the agent on the individual patient. For this reason, nurses should be attentive to the dosage given and should observe carefully the behavior manifestations and physical condition. Both accurate reporting and recording of these observations will facilitate effective adjustment of the prescribed therapy according to the patient's needs. Any sensitivity or toxic reaction should be reported immediately since some reactions can be of serious consequence.

It is not unusual to find that patients complain of loss of appetite and nausea, particularly at the start of the drug therapy. Attention should be given to the patient's symptoms which may indicate adjustments in food and their preparation. A dry mouth and a peculiar taste may indicate the preferred use of liquids to solids. If constipation is also a problem, fluids and roughage should be abundant in the diet. An accurate report of the nutritional intake is essential to protect physical stamina. In many cases these patients develop a lowered resistance to disease and are prone to upper respiratory infections.

Drowsiness is also a reaction which frequently accompanies the beginning of therapy. It is not unusual to find that the patients are sleepy, slow moving, and lack initiative to do anything. In many instances this effect is transient; however, the patient should be given reassurance and an explanation to allay his fears. Some patients may need encouragement to participate in ward activities and some may have difficulty in maneuvering safely. At such times, they should be allowed to rest in bed or a chair. Lightheadedness and weakness sometimes accompany drowsiness and may be signs of hypotension. Careful observation and good judgment are important in this phase of therapy.

The sedentary routine and the remanents of custodial care which unfortunately persist in many hospitals are being disrupted by the changes which the use of the ataraxics is effecting. Patients whose agitated, disturbed behavior held a fear and threat to personnel and those whose behavior tended to blend them with the institutional walls in the eyes of personnel cannot be ignored any longer. Unfortunately, there are patients who still remain unchanged by these aids; however, they are fewer in number.

The incorporation of drugs as a part of psychiatric treatment has not only necessitated a change in routine but has also opened new avenues for nurse-patient relationships. Attention to ways and means of strengthening nurse-patient, patient-patient relationships should be part of the plan in the rehabilitation process.

Patients who, without drugs, were unapproachable may now be amenable and accessible to personnel and the environment. Psychiatrists, nurses, and other personnel should work cooperatively in establishing an environment conducive to improvement. The supportive therapies (occupational, recreational, music, and educational) should be utilized to the patients' advantage. With this increased need for personnel who participate, the nurse should consider a plan to teach and assist untrained personnel to work cooperatively with the nurses. The nurse, in turn, needs to consider a plan which rehabilitates the patient toward a more normal existence within the hospital and eventually in the home and community.

Perhaps the most bewildered people in this whole sequence of events are the patients' families. Many are being called upon to assume responsibility for their relative patients. The nurse will be called upon to explain the patient's change, after years of unapproachable behavior. She may be the innocent recipient of the family's hostility which stems from guilt feelings, fear, or frustration. She has a very important role to play in helping the family to help her patient. Although this has been mentioned before, the drugs and their effect have made this responsibility more vital.

The large number of patients who have been returned to their community has created much interest on the part of the public in general. The nurse has an important role to play in the education and reassurance of the public. The acceptance by the community of the improved patient would contribute vastly to his recovery.

References

Behnken, Priscilla B., and Merrill, Elizabeth G.: Nursing care following prefrontal lobotomy, American Journal of Nursing 49:431-434, July 1949.

Berblinger, Klaus W.: The influence of personalities on drug therapy, American Journal of Nursing 59:1130-1132, Aug. 1959.

Bidder, G.: Are drugs the answer in mental depression? American Journal of Nursing 61:60-63, Oct. 1961.

Bombard, Pauline L., and Stevens, Leonard F.: A prefrontal lobotomy program, American Journal of Nursing 49:749-753, Dec. 1949.

Bross, Robert B.: The modern mood-changing drugs, American Journal of Nursing 57:1142-1143, 1146, Sept. 1957.

Bueker, Kathleen: Group therapy in a new setting, American Journal of Nursing 57:1581-1585, Dec. 1957.

Clawson, Gertrude: Nursing care of psychiatric patients receiving insulin therapy; For patients who are ambulatory during treatment, American Journal of Nursing 49:621-623, Oct. 1949.

Freeman, Walter, Watts, James, and Ewald, Florence: Psychosurgery: The nursing problem, American Journal of Nursing 47:210-213, April 1947.

Freeman, Walter: Psychosurgery. In Arieti, Silvana, editor: American handbook of psychiatry, New York, 1959, Basic Books, Inc., vol. 2, pp. 1521-1540.

Gelber, Ida: Tranquilizers help in posthospital care of mental patients, Nursing World 133:17-20, Nov. 1959.

Gordon, Hirsch L.: The new chemotherapy in mental illness, New York, 1958, Philosophical Library, Inc.

Hoch, Paul: Drug therapy. In Arieti, Silvana, editor: American handbook of psychiatry, New York, 1959, Basic Books, Inc., vol. 2, pp. 1541-1551.

Horwitz, William A.: Insulin shock therapy. In Arieti, Silvana, editor: American handbook of psychiatry, New York, 1959, Basic Books, Inc., vol. 2, pp. 1485-1498.

Kalinowsky, Lothar B.: Convulsive shock treatment. In Arieti, Silvana, editor: American handbook of psychiatry, New York, 1959, Basic Books, Inc., vol. 2, pp. 1499-1520.

Kalinowsky, L. B., and Hoch, P. H.: Somatic treatments in psychiatry, New York, 1961, Grune & Stratton, Inc.

Lynn, Frances H., and Friedhoff, Arnold J.: The patient on a tranquilizing regime, American Journal of Nursing 60:234-240, Feb. 1960.

McGraw, Robert B., and Oliven, John F.: Miscellaneous therapy. In Arieti, Silvana, editor: American handbook of psychiatry, New York, 1959, Basic Books, Inc., vol. 2, pp. 1552-1582.

Maloney, Elizabeth M., and Johannesen, Lucile: How the tranquilizers affect nursing practice, American Journal of Nursing 57:1144-1147, Sept. 1957.

Morgan, Moiveline M., and Denny, Mary F.: Retraining after a prefrontal lobotomy, American Journal of Nursing 55:59-62, Jan. 1955.

Noyes, Arthur P., and Kolb, Lawrence C.: Modern clinical psychiatry, ed. 6, Philadelphia, 1963, W. B. Saunders Co., pp. 524-555.

Peasley, Edgar L.: Nursing care of psychiatric patients receiving insulin therapy; For patients having coma shock treatment, American Journal of Nursing 49:623-626, Oct. 1949.

Organic behavior disorders

Chapter XVII

Characteristics of organic
behavior disorders

The ability to function adequately as a social being is dependent upon the possession of an organic equilibrium which makes organization of behavior possible. In particular, the five senses and the central nervous system permit the individual to be aware of his environment, to interpret it and its significance including his own relationship to it, and to behave in response to environmental stimuli in a manner that is appropriate. The disorganization that is characteristic of behavior disorders may be precipitated by organic damage which leaves the individual with reduced powers to cope with his surroundings. The invasion of the cortex of the frontal lobes by the spirochete of syphilis, with resultant death of nerve cells, may interfere markedly with the ability to retain and recall experience. In turn this is likely to produce anxiety since it makes the correct interpretation of the environment difficult and behavior less appropriate and effective. The less effective behavior calls forth repercussions from the environment and adds to the anxiety. Interestingly enough, the resulting pattern of behavior disorder is more closely related to the patient's basic personality than to the degree or location of the somatic pathologic changes. It would probably be correct to look upon the organic damage as the precipitating factor in the development of the behavior disorder.

Organically induced behavior disorders fall into two broad groups: acute reactions which usually develop in a toxic setting and chronic reactions which are insidious in onset and progressive in nature. The acute type tends to be reversible so that complete recovery is a good possibility. The chronic reactions have a poor ultimate prognosis as a rule since the disease processes involved result in the complete destruction of nerve cells which cannot be replaced. If the disease is one in which treatment can be effective, as in syphilis, early treatment can grant a good prognosis in chronic organic types, but if the disease is a progressive one for which no treatment is known, as in senility, the probable outcome is a steadily downhill course until death intervenes.

Organic behavior disorders may and often do present types of behavior which fall into the categories previously discussed as functional. In addition to this, there are the signs and symptoms of the organic processes peculiar to the disease involved. The type of symptoms in this group of disorders is related to the loss of function, to the patient's basic personality, and to the patient's reaction to his illness.

The signs of loss of function reflect the specific part of the nervous system that is damaged, but certain generalizations are frequently applicable. Intellectual capacity is usually reduced and is reflected in emotional instability and loss of social sensitivity caused by poor judgment. Memory defects occur, and recent memory is first and most deeply affected. Although it is not totally accurate, remote memory is a little better, and many patients show a tendency to live in the past and reminisce a great deal. The grasp of current events is usually inadequate, and because of the memory defect and poor evaluation of the present, confabulation is used to fill in the gaps. Disorientation in all three spheres—place, person, and time—is common, and the patient cannot accurately identify himself, his location, or the date.

Along with the intellectual deterioration, emotional instability and explosiveness are common occurrences. Patients with pathologic disease of the brain tend to overrespond quickly on inadequate stimulus. The emotional outburst is of brief duration, and shifting moods are typical. The general emotional trend is usually related to the premorbid personality, and individuals who were aggressive, for example, remain predominantly so. The particular additional mood variants that are most likely to be added to the basic pattern are irritability and suspiciousness. This is understandable as a reaction of the patient to his failing adequacy, for which he must seek an explanation.

The lack of judgment that goes with reduced intellectual capacity brings about behavior that conflicts with accepted social standards. Habit deterioration occurs, and ethic standards are sometimes rather flagrantly offended. It is usually some episode of this nature that brings the patient's difficulty to the attention of persons about him. Ordinarily, the previous social history will show adequate judgment, and the patient's change in behavior points up his need for help.

Symptoms in the areas of intellectual, emotional, and social inadequacy are accompanied by the signs and symptoms of neurologic or somatic illness. For example, pupillary changes, positive colloidal gold curve in the spinal fluid, inability to calculate, tremors, positive blood and spinal Wassermann tests, and other findings are present in parenchymatous syphilis. Tumors that impinge on the cerebral cortex may be fairly well located by electroencephalography. Epilepsy may be diagnosed by grand mal and petit mal convulsive features in conjunction with electroencephalography. Paralysis and muscular weakness may identify the occurrence and location of a cerebral accident. In any instance, there will be a pattern of signs and symptoms to indicate the particular type of organic damage that is present.

The basic personality of the patient determines the kind of behavior disorder he will develop. Exaggeration of the basic personality trends is common since emotional conflicts and repressed experiences tend to come to the surface as the patient's behavior becomes disorganized and previously maintained controls are weakened. A withdrawn, reserved person will most likely show a withdrawn behavior disorder. A suspicious individual will probably show a projective behavior disorder. It is not the exact location or the extent of the somatic disorder that will determine the type of behavior disorder the patient presents, but rather the premorbid personality.

The reaction of the patient to his illness is quite significant since the behavior disorder is not a necessary corollary of any disease that involves the central nervous system, any more than it is an inevitable accompaniment of pneumonia or heart disease. The patient can compensate for his failings and inadequacies and learn to live with them. Senile changes in the brain structure do not always mean senile psychosis. A great deal can be accomplished by a psychotherapeutic approach to the problems presented by the organic behavior disorder through recognizing the importance of the patient's reaction to his illness as a major factor in the resulting behavior disorder and using the knowledge to help the patient accept and live with his reduced mental capacity. Psychotherapy is as important in the treatment of syphilis of the central nervous system as chemotherapy.

The typical course of events differs in the acute and chronic forms of organic behavior disorders. The acute organic reactions are usually the result of a toxic condition which produces generalized edema of the brain. The toxin may be the result of a disease process anywhere in the body, or it may be the result of a drug or other outside agent introduced into the body. A delirious episode in infectious diseases was a common occurrence before the recent development of effective antibiotics and in many instances went along with a high temperature from any cause. Meningitis, pneumonia, and cardiorenal infections no longer, as a rule, produce deliria because of prompt and adequate treatment. Even the acute reaction of delirium tremens in excessive drinkers can frequently be aborted through prompt administration of intravenous glucose and insulin. The delirium as such has lost much of its terror for the health professions. It is most commonly seen today in response to drugs which have a cumulative effect in persons who unwisely take overdoses of bromides, barbiturates, and the like. The acute reaction also occurs following head trauma and as an incident in the course of chronic organic psychosis.

The acute organic reaction may vary markedly in depth from a mild confusion to delirium, stupor, and coma. It may progress through all of those stages, and if the patient recovers, he may experience all of these reactions in reverse in the process of recovery. It is characterized by gross disorientation, poor retention, inadequate grasp of events, and other signs of pathologic changes in the central nervous system. When confused, the patient is restless and irritable, his attention span is limited, he misidentifies people and misinterprets what happens, his conversation loses coherence, and he shows defects in recent memory and immediate recall. As the confusion increases and delirium appears, continuity of behavior is completely lost. The confusion and disorientation increase, tremors develop, restlessness mounts, insomnia becomes marked, and hallucinations and delusions dominate and determine behavior. Hallucinations are most often visual or tactile and produce anxiety and fear. Both hallucinations and delusions are related to past experience, of course, and the delirium may center around occupational habits. There may be brief lucid intervals in almost any period of the delirium. If the condition is progressive, the patient next begins to show a general reduction in activity that increases until stupor is present, and then coma may occur. The illness may terminate in a matter of hours, days, or weeks at any stage—confusion, delirium, stupor, or coma. Prompt and adequate detoxification of the patient may influence the course of events. Complete recovery without residual cerebral incompetence is always a good possibility and depends upon the nature of the toxic agent and the length of time before the patient can be rid of it. The psychotic episode can persist beyond the length of time it is organically justified, in which case the outcome depends upon adequate psychotherapy and the patient's personality resources.

In contrast to the acute organic behavior disorders in which the patient is relatively suddenly overwhelmed with a massive behavior disorganization that is striking, chronic or progressive disorders usually begin slowly and insidiously and show a steady or intermittent downhill course. Instead of a rising crescendo of symptoms that terminate in death or recovery in a limited time, the patient shows increasing memory defect, diminishing adaptive ability, and increasing signs of cerebral pathologic changes. The slowness of the process may permit him to remain in society without treatment for a longer period of time than is good for him or for his family.

One of the first symptoms to be noticed is a defect in recent memory. The patient becomes increasingly forgetful. He cannot remember where he puts things, he tells the same story over and over again to the same person, he cannot retain new experiences, and he is confused by new situations. Since remote memory is better retained at first, he places present events in the past and past events in the present. He leans on the past more and more heavily, and he becomes less and less effective in the present.

Beginning with the memory defect, there is a progressive loss of ability to function effectively in social situations. The reduced mental capacity produces loss of judgment and loss of the ability to predict the consequences of any act and thereby control behavior. The patient is less controlled by social standards and grows careless in personal appearance. Sudden impulses are indulged thoughtlessly, and behavior with an immoral connotation may be evident. Sexual offenses with small children, sexual promiscuity, or exhibitionism may occur. Emotional instability is often shown by excessive or inappropriate emotional responses. Language, behavior, thinking, and symbolic skills which are essential to communication with others will be eventually affected, and when they are, the maintenance of continuity of behavior becomes almost impossible. The downhill course may go on until the patient leads a vegetative existence in which only stereotyped responses remain.

The organic behavior disorders are precipitated by a loss or destruction of the organic matrix, which is the foundation of behavior. Their treatment and care are based on the twofold approach of stemming or repairing the organic defect and helping the patient to adjust to his reduced capacities.

References

Cameron, Norman: The psychology of behavior disorders, Boston, 1947, Houghton Mifflin Co., pp. 540-575.

Noyes, Arthur P., and Kolb, Lawrence C.: Modern clinical psychiatry, ed. 6, Philadelphia, 1963, W. B. Saunders Co., pp. 65-67, 142-145.

Chapter XVIII

Nursing care of patients with acute organic behavior disorders

The majority of acute organic behavior disorders are the result of a toxic reaction caused by a disease process within the body, such as infection, or by toxins introduced into the body, such as bromides or barbiturates. Any substance which interferes with the metabolic efficiency of the organism is potentially capable of producing a toxic state.

Toxic reactions

The toxic reaction, characterized particularly by delirium, shows consistently the postmortem finding of brain edema in all instances in which an autopsy has been possible. It is believed that the severity of the delirium may be related to the degree of brain edema.

The course of the reaction is initiated with confusion and impairment of consciousness. The patient becomes restless, does not correctly interpret his environment, shows a recent memory defect, and is disoriented. Hallucinations frequently occur, and the patient's behavior is strongly influenced by them. The hallucinations, misinterpretation, and misunderstanding of the environment produce an emotional response of fear and apprehension. Although the patient's behavior may appear bizarre and inappropriate, it is frequently not so when it is understood in relation to the hallucinations. The patient may be trying to escape from threats against himself and may attempt to jump out a window. He may persistently try to get out of bed because he thinks it is full of insects or animals. In any case the patient's seemingly irrational behavior is related to the disordered content of his thinking. In view of this fact, the patient should always be considered a potential danger to himself and to his environment.

Although fear and apprehension are the predominant mood characteristics, the mood also shows lability and irritability in rapid flashes. Speech may become rambling and incoherent, and in severe stages may consist of muttering which is completely unintelligible. Stupor or coma may finally appear and death may result. Although they almost always precede death, stupor and coma do not always presage its occurrence.

Physically the patient looks acutely ill. Vasomotor instability is shown in flushing, pallor, excessive perspiration, rapid pulse, and fluctuating blood pressure. Respirations show a deviation from normal. The temperature fluctuates and may be either very high or very low, depending on the toxin and the patient's response. Tremors of the fingers, hands, lips, and facial muscles are common. During lucid intervals the patient complains of headache and weakness.

Toxins which can produce the described syndrome are numerous. Overdoses of barbiturates, prolonged ingestion of bromides which accumulate in the bloodstream, and heavy metals such as lead and mercury acquired through occupational exposure are examples. Infectious diseases which cause a high temperature, toxemia, and exhaustion are also accompanied by delirium. Pneumonia, cardiorenal disease, acute nephritis, rheumatic fever, and malaria are examples.

Treatment of such reactions is based upon detoxification and then rehabilitation of the patient's personality, if this is indicated. A patient whose toxic condition is caused by occupational exposure to industrial poisons may present no or few problems in rehabilitation unless there is a residual reduction of physical or intellectual ability. On the other hand, a patient whose toxic condition is produced by reliance on the continual use of bromides or barbiturates to help him through his emotional crises is definitely in need of personality rehabilitation to enable him to discard his emotional crutches.

The process of detoxification is adjusted to the nature of the particular toxin. In bromide poisoning, for example, large doses of sodium chloride are indicated since the chloride ion replaces the bromide ion and makes its elimination from the body easier. Fluid intake should be increased and elimination vigorously promoted. Intensive vitamin therapy is used to promote the metabolic efficiency of the body. Since the function of the brain is related to adequate carbohydrate metabolism, the administration of intravenous glucose and insulin is frequently indicated. Sedation is avoided if possible, but if needed, it is used cautiously, and full consideration is given to the chemical nature of the offending toxin. Careful supervision of the patient during the delirious period is necessary to protect him from injury and to allay his apprehension. The environment should be as nonstimulating as possible.

Once the acute stage is over and the patient is relatively free of toxin, reassurance in regard to the episode is usually needed. Rehabilitation is directed toward self-understanding and self-acceptance in order that the patient may be able to get along with handicaps acquired during the illness or may learn to adjust without reliance on the use of toxins.

Traumatic psychoses

An acute reaction may occur in response to a head injury which, incidentally, does not always mean brain injury. A severe enough blow may produce mild confusion, with intellectual dulling, amnesia for a brief period, and mild ataxia without resulting in unconsciousness. The usual outcome is rapid with complete recovery unless the incident happens to be a precipitating factor in the development of a behavior disorder in a susceptible individual. Trauma to the head and brain may be severe enough to immediately produce unconsciousness. As recovery takes place, the patient is ordinarily confused, dull, and ataxic when he becomes conscious, and in some instances he may show a typical delirious reaction such as previously described. Such a reaction is an exception rather than a rule and its occurrence has not yet been demonstrated to be related to the extent or location of the brain injury. Traumatic brain injury may also leave permanent residuals which result in impaired performance of the individual as a person.

Nursing care

The nursing care of patients with acute organic reactions requires a blending of the arts of medical and psychiatric nursing. The use of one without the other complicates the picture in both areas. Poor medical care increases the psychiatric problem, and poor psychiatric care increases the medical problem.

Psychotherapeutic environment. The patient with acute cerebral incompetence needs an environment in which control of both the patient and the environment is possible. Because he is a potential danger to himself and his environment, the patient needs constant observation. Since restraint produces apprehension and fear, particularly in persons who are unable to grasp and understand current events adequately, there must be someone readily available to prevent the patient from getting out of bed, trying to jump out of the window, assaulting other persons, or otherwise endangering himself or other persons. Since the patient is apprehensive and tends to misinterpret his environment, stimulation should be reduced to a minimum. In connection with this, it must be remembered that sensitivity to the meaning of experience to the patient is necessary to reduce stimulation effectively. If, for example, a toxic patient sees frogs jumping from a picture on the wall, the picture may be removed. Whenever possible the particular sources of stimulation to the patient should be carefully analyzed, and an attempt should be made to reduce stimulation from that source. The essence of a therapeutic environment for an acutely toxic patient consists of three elements: the necessary physical equipment for care, reduction of stimuli to which the patient is sensitive, and adequate protection for the patient.

Interpersonal relationships. Interpersonal needs of an acutely toxic patient center primarily around his apprehension and fear. Constant reassurance in a firm and positive manner is necessary, along with the realization that reassurance will need almost constant repetition because of clouded sensorium, disorientation, and memory defect. If the patient fears insects in his bed, he should be assured there are none. A brief demonstration may be given, and a positive declaration that the fear will soon disappear should be made. This should be repeated as often as necessary without impatience or irritation. When the patient is indecisive, decisions should be made quickly and firmly for him.

Considerable ingenuity is required to secure the cooperation of the patient with necessary physical measures, and force should be avoided if possible. Full advantage may be taken of the patient's memory defect, distractibility, and short attention span. Lucid intervals should be watched for, recognized, and treated as such.

So far as possible it is wise to limit the number of persons to whom the patient is exposed during the acute period. The same nurses, day after day, familiar with the patient's psychotic content and reactions, can reduce to a minimum the threats the environment may carry for the patient.

Physical needs. The patient in a toxic delirious state needs constant nursing care directed toward physical comfort and elimination of the offending toxin. Fluids should be forced, but it should be kept in mind that this must be accompanied by increased elimination since an increase in fluid in the tissues may well tend to increase brain edema. Accurate records of intake and output should be kept. Skin care is important since the patient perspires profusely and is likely to be restless, thus increasing the danger of skin breaks and infections. A bath is needed more often than once a day, bed linen should be changed often to keep the patient clean and comfortable, and drafts (to which the patient is susceptible) should be avoided. Particular attention should be paid to physical comfort through such measures as attention to oral hygiene, bed linen kept smooth, pillows adjusted to the patient's comfort, and adequate ventilation of the room.

As soon as possible the patient should be encouraged to eat, and an intake high in both vitamins and calories is indicated. Fluids should continue to be forced until the patient's toxic condition is past.

Any signs or symptoms that would indicate focal areas of cerebral embarrassment should be promptly reported. The presence of unequal pupils or an indication of paralysis or hyperesthesia constitute examples.

Since the patient needs constant physical attention, the nurse should carry out procedures as quietly and efficiently as possible, making every effort to secure the patient's cooperation in order to avoid stimulation. Quiet reassurance should mark everything the nurse does for the patient. Indecisiveness should be avoided because it may upset the patient, who needs an environment on which he can completely depend.

Protection. A delirious patient needs someone to accept complete responsibility for him. In his confused state he is incapable of protecting himself from injury or of being aware of injury caused to others if he becomes assaultive. The things and persons he fears should be thoroughly known to those persons who care for him, and he should be carefully protected from injury. Sideboards may be necessary to keep him from falling out of bed, the bed may need to be well away from windows or doors, and the patient should have assistance if he is out of bed for any reason.

Group relations. During the delirious state, the patient's contacts with other people should be as limited as possible. When the patient is up and about, he should be encouraged to join other patients and should be permitted to freely exchange experiences if he wishes. Because of the relative intellectual clearness that accompanies the recovery from a toxic period, even in acutely psychotic patients, the patient may well be a valuable group member. Any tendency to withdraw or stay alone should be discouraged. It is particularly important to establish group contacts as early as possible if the patient is left with a residual handicap.

Convalescence. During the convalescent period, much will depend upon the type of toxic infection, the residual handicap, if any, and the patient's basic personality. Problems will be related to these three factors, and their balance will indicate the points of emphasis. If the patient has been dependent upon the use of toxins to adjust, he will need encouragement to develop independence and to accept his illness without leaning on it as an alibi or a means to gain sympathy. If the patient is left with some permanent brain damage, he will need help in accepting his new limitation. Careful study of the patient to help him effectively use his strengths and to improve or accept his weaknesses is indicated.

The convalescent period should not bore the patient with inactivity nor tire him out. An interesting occupation adjusted to his physical ability is important in shortening the period of recovery to full strength. The attitude of personnel toward the patient's illness should avoid either ridicule or criticism. The temptation to show amusement concerning the patient's inappropriate or bizarre behavior during the acute phase should be carefully assessed against his genuine feeling about the matter. Few persons like to be laughed at, even though they may pretend they do.

References

Cohen, Sidney, and Klein, Hazel K.: The delirious patient, American Journal of Nursing **58**:685-687, May 1958.

Ebaugh, Franklin G., and Tiffany, William J., Jr.: Infective-exhaustive psychoses. In Arieti, Silvana, editor: American handbook of psychiatry, New York, 1959, Basic Books, Inc., vol. 2, pp. 1231-1248.

Levin, Max: Toxic psychoses. In Arieti, Silvana, editor: American handbook of psychiatry, New York, 1959, Basic Books, Inc., vol. 2, pp. 1222-1230.

Noyes, Arthur P., and Kolb, Lawrence C.; Modern clinical psychiatry, ed. 6, Philadelphia, 1963, W. B. Saunders Co., pp. 145-163, 182-193.

Chapter XIX

Nursing care of patients with
chronic organic behavior disorders

Some of the more important progressive organic behavior disorders are summarized briefly as examples before the nursing care for patients with chronic organic behavior disorders is presented.

Senile psychoses

Behavior disorders in the senile psychoses are caused by changes accompanying old age which result in an increasing inability to adjust and to adapt to the environment. The brain shrinks, and the cortical areas atrophy, with a loss of cells and areas of destruction called senile plaques (which can be demonstrated microscopically) are formed. Fat is markedly increased throughout the brain. Reflecting the loss of functioning cortical cells, the patient shows behavior changes to which he may or may not be able to adapt.

The usual onset of a senile behavior disorder is so gradual that it is often not recognized until some rather startling or shocking failure on the part of the patient calls it sharply into focus. The patient shows increasing forgetfulness and disturbance in orientation. As the patient's grasp of current events begins to slip because of difficulties with retention and recall, interests narrow and new ideas and activities are more difficult to accept. Habits become both more rigid and more deteriorated. Caution becomes suspiciousness, and orderliness becomes compulsiveness. The poorer contact results in a reduced capacity to respond with habits of personal cleanliness. Mood becomes labile, and the capacity for depth and continuity of affection for others is reduced and may eventually be lost. The course of the illness is progressive, and intellectual ability may become so impaired that the patient retains merely a few stereotyped responses from his past experience. He will then exist on a vegetative level until death occurs.

The form of behavior displayed when the patient becomes psychotic will express the basic personality plus his reaction to his failing abilities. The reaction may be predominantly aggressive, depressive, projective, agitated, or withdrawn, depending on the individual. In any instance the behavior will not be specific for the cerebral areas involved.

Treatment for patients with senile changes is aimed primarily at helping the patient accept his reduced capacities through psychotherapy and, when possible, by reducing environmental demands and threats. The course is a steadily progressive one, and the cerebral damage that occurs is not reversible.

Behavior disorders with cerebral arteriosclerosis

In cerebral arteriosclerosis also, behavior disorders occur as the result of an inadequate blood supply to the brain that impairs effective function of cerebral cells. Since arteriosclerosis occurs in persons in the same age group as persons with senile reactions and since the same somatic areas are involved, arteriosclerotic patients present much the same type of illness. For all practical purposes the only differences are a somewhat more acute onset, a tendency to periodic remissions, a greater personal awareness of physical changes in the early stages, and the occurrence of cerebral accidents in arteriosclerotic patients. Otherwise the general picture of increasing cerebral incompetence, plus the patient's reaction to it, is present.

Medical procedures designed to lower blood cholesterol have been employed in the treatment of cerebral arteriosclerosis, but their value has been controversial. Reduction in cholesterol and a cholesterol-free diet have been tried, and thyroid, iodides, cortisone, and ACTH have been administered. Nicotinic acid and nicotinamide do seem to improve cerebral circulation. Other measures that are used include shock therapy for depressions and agitations and group therapy as an aid in adjustment to limited abilities.

Senile and cerebral arteriosclerotic behavior disorders have become an important social problem in recent years. The increasing life expectancy has kept alive a greater number of people to succumb to the particular difficulties of old age. The trend toward urbanization of the population has added to the problem since urban life offers greater hazards to the aged, and the pattern of life in cities makes less provision for them than does that of life in rural areas. Social facilities adapted to the needs of older persons have not yet been developed, and as a result large numbers of them are finding their way into state psychiatric hospitals.

General paresis

General paresis is a syphilitic infection of the meninges and encephalon and is most marked in the cerebral cortex of the frontal and parietal regions. Why some patients develop syphilis of the central nervous system, whereas others do not, is a moot question.

The serologic and neurologic findings in general paresis are nearly always adequate for diagnosis. Neurologically, pupillary changes occur, and the pupils may be unequal, dilated, or contracted. The Argyll Robertson

pupil, which reacts to accommodation but not to light, is a common finding. Progressive weakness and incoordination of voluntary muscles is shown
in tremors of the tongue, hands, and face, in disturbance of speech, especially slurring, and in changes in handwriting. The lack of coordination of tongue muscles is shown in the patient's inability to enunciate
accurately such test phrases as "Methodist Episcopal" and "Third riding
artillery brigade." Deep tendon reflexes are affected and may be exaggerated, diminished, or lost. Because of the nerve cell damage, the facial
muscles may be relaxed and smoothed out, resulting in a younger but
somewhat vacant expression.

Serologically, the blood and spinal Wassermann tests may be positive
if the patient's syphilitic infection has not been treated. Spinal fluid pressure is usually increased, lymphocytes and proteins are well above normal limits, and globulin is present in the spinal fluid. The Lange colloidal
gold curve shows positive findings.

In regard to the behavior aspect, the early symptoms are usually slowing of the mental processes, memory defect, irritability, and increasing
loss of judgment and social skills. As the disease progresses, the organic
indications of reduced intellectual capacity become more obvious, and
the behavior disorder that follows will be in accordance with the patient's
personality and experience. He may be expansive and elated, or he may
be agitated and depressed. The form of the behavior deviation that develops is specific for the patient but not for general paresis.

Prompt and adequate treatment of general paresis may halt the disease
at any stage and prevent further damage. Treatment undertaken in the
early inflammatory stages of the infection before actual degeneration of
cortical cells has occurred may result in complete recovery for the patient. The earlier treatment is instituted, the greater the organic equipment
the patient may retain. By way of caution, not all patients respond to
treatment although the majority of them do. Nor is the complete physical
recovery of the patient an absolute guarantee that the behavior disorder
will disappear. The behavior disorder may outlast the illness which precipitated it.

By far the most effective treatment of general paresis is intensive
penicillin therapy. Recovery and improvement rates are much higher
than with older therapies such as induced malaria. Large doses of penicillin, up to 15 to 20 million units, are indicated. The treatment is effective,
rapid, inexpensive, and carries practically no risk.

Behavior disorders with convulsions

Convulsive phenomena may occur as a symptom of cerebral irritation
in organic brain disease or in any illness which affects the central nervous
system. Thus it may be a symptom of paresis, meningitis, cerebral arteriosclerosis, uremia, lead poisoning, or any other toxic condition. Convulsive
phenomena are also an indication of idiopathic or essential epilepsy. The
actual convulsions or their equivalents occur as evidence of the disordered

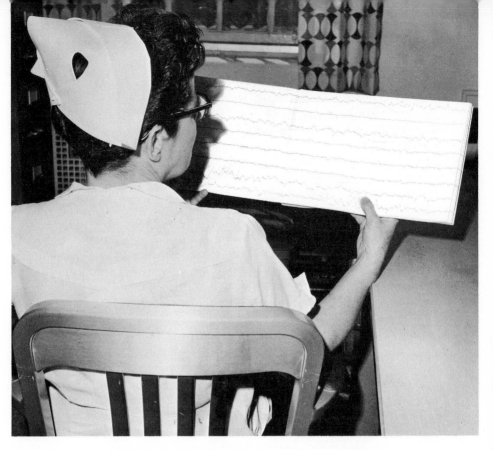

Electroencephalogram recordings provide a source of information about the electric activity of the patient's brain.

function of the rate-regulating mechanism of the brain. Electric currents are produced in the brain, and the electric discharge takes place at a regular rhythmic rate ordinarily. During the period of a convulsion or its substitute, the epileptic patient shows a marked variation in the rate of discharge as measured by the electroencephalograph. What happens during a convulsion is known, but what initiates the event is unknown.

Epilepsy occurs as a grand mal, petit mal, or psychomotor episode although a patient not uncommonly shows a mixture of types. All are characterized by a disturbance in consciousness. A grand mal seizure follows a definite pattern. An aura or warning may or may not occur, but is usually specific for the individual patient and is related to one of the five senses. The patient may see a bright light or a vision, hear something, smell a peculiar smell, or experience some indication that an attack is on the way. The convulsion is initiated with a tonic spasm involving the entire body and is accompanied by a loss of consciousness. The body is then involved in a series of jerking motions, lasting one-half to a whole minute or slighty more. The convulsion is followed by a period of stupor of varying length, and confusion ordinarily accompanies the return to consciousness. A petit mal attack is a momentary loss of consciousness often accompanied by localized muscular twitching. The loss of consciousness is so brief that the patient does not fall. Psychomotor attacks, or epileptic equivalents, cover a variety of types of behavior, including episodes of overactivity, furors of violent frenzy, and periods of amnesia. Patients with convulsive disorders can and do lead perfectly normal lies and adjust well to their handicap. Some of them, however, do require institutionalization and some show severe behavior disorders. The behavior disorders center around (1) mood disturbances marked by ill humor, cruelty, sickly sentimentality, and marked emotional lability, (2) periods of confusion which may include hallucinatory experiences, and (3) deterioration. Whether the deterioration is a result of the disease, the medication given for the disease, or the social isolation that all too often accompanies epilepsy is uncertain. Fortunately a psychotic development in the course of epilepsy is the exception rather than the rule.

The treatment of behavior disorders with convulsive phenomena is based on medication to control seizures, regulation of diet, and environmental adjustment. Phenobarbital, Dilantin Sodium, Mesantoin, and Mysoline are commonly used in the treatment of grand mal and psychomotor attacks. Tridione, Paradione, and Milontin are administered in the treatment of petit mal attacks. Dosage is very much an individual matter and must be worked out for each patient.

Huntington's chorea

Huntington's chorea is a rare form of behavior disorder for two reasons. First, its occurrence is not common, and, second, it is one illness that is nearly always accompanied by incapacitating behavior changes in which heredity can be demonstrated as the chief etiologic factor. It reveals its presence in middle age and results from gradual degeneration of specific areas in the brain. The physical symptoms are quite striking. Jerky, clumsy, and irregular movements, beginning in the upper extremities and slowly but surely involving the entire body, render the patient quite conspicuous as well as unable to carry out normal activities. Understandably, the patient becomes irritable, emotionally labile, and quite suspicious. Attention, memory, and judgment become quite impaired. Custodial detention usually becomes necessary as dementia progresses.

Postencephalitic behavior disorders

Epidemic encephalitis, a virus disease, takes as many forms as a chameleon and often has a residual in postencephalitic behavior disorders. At one time Parkinson's syndrome was believed to be a belated result of the acute form of epidemic encephalitis, as well as being due to other causes. As the acute form has no very specific course, so the residual behavior disorder has no specific form when it does occur. Any inflammatory disease of the brain may precipitate a behavior disorder of almost any hue and may also leave chronic brain inflammation or damage that may precipitate a behavior disorder. One of the most interesting is Parkinson's syndrome, which is characterized by listlessness, avoidance of experience, masklike facies, and typical pill-rolling movements of the fingers. In Parkinson's syndrome, the patient presents a typical physical appearance which is of importance in precipitating a behavior disorder. The involuntary or smooth muscle is tensed, and the resultant appearance and behavior show drooling, slow and monotonous speech, and slow and shuffling gait, with the trunk bent forward and arms flexed before the trunk. The thumbs and finger combine in a characteristic pill-rolling motion. A tremor of the fingers, hands, feet, and head develops progressively. This shaking palsy with its marked intention tremor is seen as a sequela to brain infections and usually produces a marked reaction in patients who undergo the experience. These symptoms will be enhanced or minimized by the patient's reaction to them. In any instance, the encephalitis of whatever origin and its sequelae are precipitating factors in a behavior disorder.

Drugs to control the physical symptoms of Parkinson's syndrome have long been used. Among the oldest, and still useful, are atropine and hyoscine. Rabellon (a combination of hyoscyamine, atropine, and scopolamine) has been effective in some persons. Parpanit and Disipal, which have atropine-like reactions, have received favorable reports. Newer drugs include Artane, Pagitane, Parsidol, Kremadin, and Diparcol.

Nursing care

The nursing care of patients with progressive cerebral incompetence offers a real challenge. Until recently the attitude toward such behavior disorders has been so completely hopeless that they have been considered an area in which little could be accomplished. A beginning realization of how much can be done in guiding the patient to live effectively and constructively with his handicap has dawned. The field is of particular interest since many behavior disorders of organic origin occcur in older persons who have previously been constructive members of society. The patients who develop behavior disorders in conjunction with progressive cerebral incompetence represent human resources well worth the effort of conservation.

Psychotherapeutic environment. The environment must be adjusted to the patient's limitations, depending on the degree of incapacitation of physical and intellectual capacities. Patients who have only a few stereotyped responses left for adaptive purposes may depend completely upon the continuity of the environment for any continuity of behavior. For such patients a routine that remains exactly the same in minute detail from day to day is essential. Progressive brain destruction tends to make it increasingly harder to cope with present and new experiences; so that increasing reliance is placed on past habits, successes, and interests. Failing abilities cause an insecurity that accentuates this trend. Therefore an important principle in environmental control for patients with chronic nervous system diseases that are accompanied by behavior disorders is careful rigidity in routine and reduction of new experiences to the lowest possible level. If the actual damage is relatively small, the patient's experience can be gradually broadened as he profits from the security of a thoroughly dependable daily routine. The patient can then be encouraged by slow steps to the highest level of activity of which he is capable.

The environment should also take into account the potential dangers in failing physical capacities such as vision, hearing, muscular coordination, etc. Although the general physical aspect should be pleasant and cheerful, furniture should be sturdy and placed where the danger of falling over it is reduced to a minimum. Extra rugs and small bits of furniture such as magazine racks and footstools should be used with caution, if not eliminated. Equipment should only be that which is essential and should be kept in the same place consistently.

Interpersonal relationships. The problems in interpersonal relationships with patients with progressive cerebral incompetence center around loss of abilities, reduced level of adaptability, and insecurity stemming from these two sources. The behavior disorder that develops, if one does, will be colored by the patient's prepsychotic personality so that the syndromes of withdrawal, aggression, projection, and preoccupation with somatic function and ritualism will also be seen. In such instances, the principles of the nursing care previously outlined for the particular type of maladjustment will be applicable.

The central objective is to build the patient's confidence and self-esteem for himself as a person with whatever handicap he has acquired. While constancy in physical environment is important, consistency in attitude and behavior toward the patient is equally essential. His routine should be tactfully manipulated until he learns to depend on it, and then encouragement toward improvement should be instituted. If the degree of intellectual impairment, the probable shortened attention span, and the potential irritability and explosive emotional response are taken into full account, the patient should be encouraged to undertake responsibilities and activities in which success is a reasonable expectation and failure a remote one. Liberal praise should be given for accomplishment and criticism avoided. Physical handicaps, such as memory defects, should not be made conspicuous nor should they be ignored. Rather, calm matter-of-fact verbal and emotional acceptance of their existence makes it easier for the patient to accept them. The patient should be helped to develop emotional control and encouraged to develop perseverance.

One area that is often a sensitive one for personnel is the patient's tendency to be less subtle than usual in regard to moral and ethical questions in both speech and behavior. The nurse should be prepared for such expressions of the loss of social skills and recognize them as symptomatic. As the patient improves in behavior, he may be helped to control this particular trait as well.

Physical needs. The physical needs of patients with progressive cere-

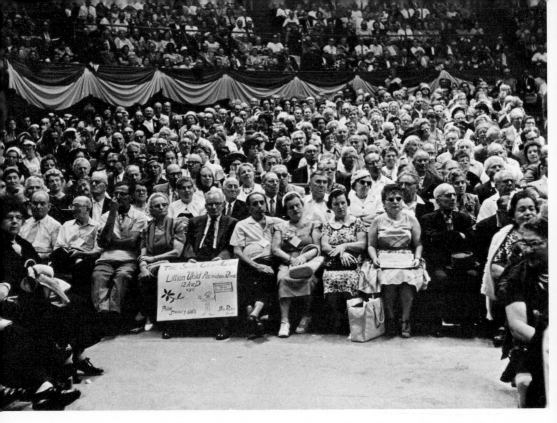

A concert and rally provides an example of community interest in the problems of senior citizens. (Courtesy Burton Berinsky, ILGWU "Justice.")

bral incompetence are numerous. Personal hygiene needs constant attention, and the establishment of health habits should be promoted. Elderly patients, for example, are frequently not too enthusiastic about a bath and change of clothing. Routine that is very much the same from day to day helps and quiet firmness is another aid. Attention should be paid to oral hygiene, skin care, elimination, and diet. It is usually not wise to attempt to change the eating habits of a lifetime, and if supplements are needed, they can be given medicinally.

Exercise adjusted to the patient's ability is a definite need. Although a patient may no longer be capable of active exercise, whatever he can do safely should be carried through. Exercise also helps with the problem of insomnia. Many patients with this type of disorder are restless at night, and to keep them interested and active in a daily routine helps them to secure adequate rest.

Convulsions do occur in diseases of the central nervous system and are common in epilepsy. When a convulsion occurs, the patient should be left where he is until the convulsion ends unless he has fallen where injury is apt to occur. If possible, something should be placed between the teeth to prevent tongue biting. Clothing should be loosened around the throat and chest, and the head should be supported to prevent injury against the floor. No attempt should be made to restrict the motion of the patient's body. When the tonic phase ends and the patient begins to breathe, the head should be turned gently to one side to prevent the aspiration of mucus which collects rapidly. At the end of the convulsion the patient is placed in a low bed, with protection against falling, and is allowed to remain until he is intellectually clear. A patient who is restless, confused, excitable, or assaultive following such an episode should be closely observed and protected from injuring himself or others. A careful and detailed descriptive report of the convulsion should be charted, including the following information: any incident preceding the convulsion, parts of the body involved, sequence of events, duration, any injury, and behavior after the convulsion.

Protective needs. The protective needs of patients with progressive cerebral incompetence tend to be rather high and are related to two factors—failing physical abilities and lack of emotional control.

Patients must be protected from self-injury caused by poor vision, poor muscular coordination, and poor memory, among other defects. Protection from drafts or extremes in temperautre, careful supervision in the bathroom to prevent falls, care in the application of heat and cold to skin surfaces, observation in the dining room to note such problems as difficulty in swallowing, and assistance up and down stairs and into and out of bed are all measures to be adopted when necessary. The nurse should be alert to the greater possibility of retention of urine and feces in patients with disorders of this type. In other words, the nurse should make herself tactfully responsible for the prevention of any injury and realize that the possibilities for such happenings are much higher than usual.

The other particular threat to the physical safety of such patients is their explosive emotional responses; assaultiveness and excited episodes are fairly common. Close observation and tactful approach, allowing the patient free verbal expression but no more, usually make the management of such episodes easier. Distractibility, poor attention span, and the briefness of such explosions can be exploited during the period of excitement. The patient should be kept away from situations which repeatedly result in difficulties.

Group relations. Patients should be encouraged to join group activities with other patients who have handicaps of similar origin. Supervision should be directed toward avoidance of failure, support when failure happens, and alertness to the possible consequences of irritability and explosiveness. The major problems usually center around getting the patient interested in activities and getting him to stay interested. Persistence pays dividends since habits can be established through consistent efforts. Patients with postencephalitic behavior disorders tend to depend more on habits than is usual.

Convalescence. Convalescent care of patients with chronic behavior disorders is usually not oriented to complete recovery but toward readjustment of the patient to his new status. Therefore, as the severity of the patient's behavior disorder subsides, the major tasks are to determine his greatest potential in terms of his probable future and to help him reach for that level and not burden himself with aspirations beyond his reach. Attaching importance to the things he can do, making them seem worth while in the eyes of others, and encouraging the development of skill in their practice will help the patient to live within his limitations. Considerable tact is required, and the single fact to keep constantly in mind is that the convalescent period should give the patient opportunity to develop skill and security in the types of activity which will constitute his life.

References

Brill, Henry: Postencephalitic psychiatric conditions. In Arieti, Silvana, editor: American handbook of psychiatry, New York, 1959, Basic Books, Inc., vol. 2, pp. 1163-1174.

Bruetsch, Walter L.: Neurosyphilitic conditions. In Arieti, Silvana, editor: American handbook of psychiatry, New York, 1959, Basic Books, Inc., vol. 2, pp. 1003-1020.

Charles, D.: Outstanding characteristics of older patients, American Journal of Nursing **61**:80, Nov. 1961.

Elliot, Alta: Parkinson's disease: Nursing care, American Journal of Nursing **55**:817-818, July 1955.

Hunscher, M.: Nutritional needs of the mentally ill geriatric patients, Journal of Psychiatric Nursing **1**:220, May 1963.

Livingston, S.: Antiepileptic drugs, American Journal of Nursing **63**:366, Oct. 1963.

Magee, Kenneth R.: Parkinson's disease: Neurological management, American Journal of Nursing **55**:814-817, July 1955.

Newberry, William B., Jr.: Sedatives have their place, but—, American Journal of Nursing **57**:1285-1286, Oct. 1957.

Newton, Kathleen: Geriatric nursing, ed. 3, St. Louis, 1960, The C. V. Mosby Co.

Noles, E.: Nursing a geriatric patient, American Journal of Nursing **63**:73, Jan. 1963.

Noyes, Arthur P., and Kolb, Lawrence C.: Modern clinical psychiatry, ed. 6, Philadelphia, 1963, W. B. Saunders Co., pp. 202-274.

Pirnie, Florence A., and Baldwin, Maitland: Observing cerebral seizures, American Journal of Nursing **59**:366-369, Mar. 1959.

Nursing care of patients who depend on emotional crutches

Chapter XX

Nursing care of patients
who depend on alcohol

The discussion of patients who depend strongly on crutches—particularly, alcohol and drugs—to enable them to cope with life has been separated from the discussion of other behavior disorders for a specific reason. Such disorders combine the features of both functional and organic disorders since current thinking about the use of alcohol and drugs places their origin in the functional disorders and some of their end stages in the organic disorders. Generally speaking, alcoholism is still considered psychogenic in origin although many attempts have been made to find some organic explanation for it. At the present, biochemical, endocrinological, and neurophysical factors in the etiology of this disorder remain obscure. The behavior disorders of persons who depend on emotional crutches are characterized by the deliberate use of an exogenous toxin introduced into the body, a toxin whose effect is to blur reality and make it more endurable.

Alcoholism constitutes a major social problem in our culture which may well be no different than it has been for preceding cultures. It has been estimated that approximately one third of the population in the United States drinks excessively, and estimates of the annual cost to society run as high as three quarters of a billion dollars. It is no secret that the American public spends more money on liquor than it spends on education.

The history of the use of alcohol dates as far back as the recorded history of man. Like many socially accepted forms of behavior, overindulgence or exaggeration in its use can become pathologic. When an individual has become so dependent upon the use of alcohol that it interferes with his success in life and he still is unable to control his drinking, he is then considered an alcoholic. The exact line where social drinking stops and alcoholism begins is extremely hard to define for any individual person.

Dependence on the consumption of alcohol is considered a symptom or a disease and may be either. Specific etiologic factors are not clearly understood. Persons who are lonely, who have feelings of inferiority, who are anxious, who have fears they cannot verbalize or identify, or who have strong passive dependent needs that are not acceptable to them may become alcoholics. Other personality characteristics generally attributed to persons with behavior disorders of this group are low tension tolerance, inability to wait for delayed satisfactions, tendency to do everything to excess, impulsiveness, and resentment toward responsibilities. However, such persons may also become withdrawn, aggressive, or neurotic. What determines the particular choice of alcohol as a method of adjustment is uncertain. Some persons drink because of social pressure and some because of inner needs. In either case, if the drinking thus started occurs in a personality with strong emotional conflicts that remain unsolved, the possibility of the development of pathologic dependence on alcohol is present.

One of the first effects of alcohol is to depress the inhibitory centers or areas in the frontal lobes and thereby reduce self-criticism and judgment and produce a more comfortable feeling of sureness and self-confidence. The reduction of inhibitory control over the self permits the free expression of strong emotions that would ordinarily be suppressed. When a person is under the influence of alcohol, deep resentment and hostility, for example, which burn him inwardly, will be openly expressed, and he will experience some relief. When he sobers up, however, tension is usually increased by the feelings of guilt and fear of retaliation that follow the expression of hostility, and alcohol becomes necessary again to release the tension. If it will be remembered, this pattern approximates one of the vicious cycles found in projective behavior disorders. In this sense alcoholic indulgence of a pathologic degree may be a symptom of basic personality maladjustment. Alcoholism may be substituted for a projective behavior disorder, may delay its appearance, or may precipitate the disorder more quickly. In the same fashion, alcoholism may be a symptom of a neurotic or psychopathic disorder or any other form of maladjustment. Alcoholism of this type may be considered secondary to the underlying disorder and is a symptom of the disorder, which is most often associated with aggressive patterns, projective patterns, and psychoneurotic and socially aggressive patterns of behavior.

The so-called disease of alcoholism develops in persons who show no characteristic premorbid personality but have difficulties in adjustment. And when they are exposed to the effect of alcohol, these persons resort to it regularly as an aid to adjustment. Such patients go on to become completely dependent upon alcohol even when its destructive effect on social adequacy becomes evident. In many instances, drinking appears compulsive in nature—the patient *must* drink and becomes increasingly tense until alcohol is available.

There is one distinction in the field that is of therapeutic significance. Individuals whose personality difficulties are obvious at an early age and whose drinking becomes a problem very early are also difficult to treat.

Individuals who have made an adequate social adjustment until 35 or 40 years of age and whose transition from social drinking to alcoholism takes place gradually at that age are much more hopeful therapeutic prospects.

The profitable effect of alcohol for persons who are uncomfortable is twofold. It both blurs the sharp edges of reality and makes the individual feel more competent to deal with reality. In persons who tolerate anxiety poorly, alcohol is a quick and effective solace. And, in the beginning, it is a socially acceptable form of behavior. However, why the alcoholic uses alcohol as an escape rather than some other defense mechanism, why he cannot stop when alcohol ceases to be a help and becomes a problem, and why he continues to drink while knowing the consequences are all unanswered questions.

The prolonged use of a toxin such as alcohol has a definite effect upon the central nervous system and its function. The immediate result of acute intoxication is well known. Motor activity is lessened and becomes poorly coordinated, speech is slurred and becomes incoherent and unintelligible, physical strength is reduced, judgment and intellectual activity are impaired, memory is less sharp, and stupor or coma may be the end result. In patients who drink constantly and heavily, a milder but chronic form of such symptoms may be seen. In fact, it may be necessary to know the person rather well to recognize the lowered motor activity, reduced physical strength, mild memory defects, and poor judgment. Prolonged use of alcohol may also produce organic behavior disorders of a rather severe form, including several variations of the acute and chronic forms.

Pathologic intoxication can occur and consists of an episode of sudden excitement usually accompanied by anger and rage, assaultiveness that may be homicidal, hallucinations, and confusion. The patient is almost always amnesic for the period and has no idea of what has occurred. Such episodes are precipitated by the ingestion of relatively small amounts of alcohol. The dynamics, either physical or psychologic, of such episodes are not understood, and they may well be wrongly classified when considered alcoholic behavior disorders.

Delirium tremens is a typical acute toxic reaction which occurs in patients who have used alcohol heavily over a prolonged period. Motor restlessness, visual hallucinations, great apprehension, marked tremors, and ataxia occur in the setting of a severe delirium. The delirium usually terminates rather abruptly in a few days.

Acute hallucinosis may occur in patients who use alcohol excessively Hallucinations, most commonly auditory, that produce extreme fear are typical features, along with an unusual retention of clearness of the sensorium. Signs of physical illness are less marked than in delirium tremens.

Korsakoff's syndrome is a chronic form of disorder in which permanent damage to the nervous system has followed prolonged and excessive drinking. Its pattern is that of a chronic organic behavior disorder. The most striking symptoms are severe memory loss and marked confabulation. As the illness progresses, there is a tendency to lose contact with reality. Peripheral neuritis or polyneuritis usually accompanies the disorder. Early and intensive treatment with vitamin B may prevent foot drop, with shuffling gait, and other neurologic complications which used to be rather common.

Chronic alcoholic deterioration occurs after years of excessive drinking which may or may not have been punctuated by episodes of hallucinatory experience or delirium tremens. Emotions become labile, suspiciousness and irritability are common, and the emotions gradually show a loss of depth. Ethical sense and judgment suffer. Evidence of an organic memory defect is finally shown, and intellectual ability deteriorates. Such patients can be included in the classification of chronic organic behavior disorders.

The treatment of alcoholic disorders has not been very profitable. Various methods of approach to the problem of therapy all seem to show good results in approximately one third of the patients treated. Recently, research and study have been intensified, and it is to be hoped that an increase in knowledge concerning alcoholism will result in better therapeutic techniques. At the present time, three broad approaches are being used although all methods have much in common.

Alcoholics Anonymous, a lay organization, has contributed a great deal to the rehabilitation of alcoholics. The founders and workers are all former alcoholics, temporarily or permanently under control, who approach alcoholic persons and offer them help. These workers prefer to call themselves more realistically, alcoholics who do not drink. The basic tenets are that the individual is unable to manage himself and needs to depend on divine help and group support in order to control his drinking, and that once he is a member of the group and under control, the individual can be a useful society member and be able to help others. Meetings are held at which experiences are freely discussed, which gives the patient both emotional catharsis and group acceptance. When and if the patient slips and begins to drink again, individual help is available during the episode from other members of the group.

A conditioned reflex method of treatment is also used and is most effective when accompanied by psychotherapy. After an intramuscular injection that produces emesis, usually emetine hydrochloride, the patient is given whiskey. The procedure is repeated until the conditioning is complete enough that the sight or smell of alcohol produces nausea and vomiting. Patients after discharge may need to return for reconditioning.

Antabuse and cortisone are also being used in the treatment of alcoholism, and Antabuse has become an effective type of therapy for some patients. Antabuse destroys the taste for alcohol, and after taking it, the patient becomes ill if alcohol is also taken. Current thinking estimates that the greatest value of Antabuse is as an adjunct in the treatment of patients who wish to control their drinking but are unable to do so without help. Cortisone is used in the treatment of acute intoxications, including delirium tremens. It brings physical symptoms under control rapidly. When

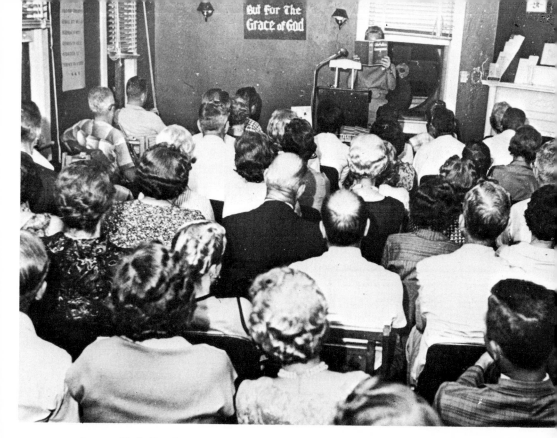

Among Alcoholics Anonymous services are meetings where alcoholic persons can discuss their problems frankly and openly.
(Courtesy General Services of Alcoholics Anonymous.)

the patient is in good physical condition, he is discharged and referred to a local unit of Alcoholics Anonymous or is treated as an outpatient for psychotherapy.

Reports on the use of tranquilizing drugs in the treatment of alcoholism are available. These drugs are particularly effective in the treatment of alcoholic delirium although they are also being used freely to help control the basic anxiety experienced by alcoholics. The most commonly used tranquilizers are derivatives of mepazine.

Psychotherapy is directed toward guiding the patient to understand himself and his problems, to face what he is trying to escape from, and to learn to live comfortably with himself as he is. He must also learn to abstain completely from the use of alcohol since most therapists are convinced that alcoholics cannot successfully stay at the level of social drinking. In order for psychotherapy to be effective, it is necessary for the patient to wish to help himself or to develop within a controlled environment the wish to help himself. Reports on treatment vary a great deal, and pessimism is rather noticeable. However, there is general agreement that treatment should not stop with the removal of the physical signs and symptoms, but must be directed toward personality rehabilitation.

Nursing care

The nursing care of patients with alcoholic behavior disorders is ordinarily as difficult as their psychiatric therapy. They are persons who tend to be charming and likeable but who do not wear well and are constantly disappointing. The situation created by constant disappointment in the patient is rife with attitude difficulties for personnel.

Psychotherapeutic environment. Because of their inability to tolerate anxiety and their customary reliance on the anxiety-solvent properties of alcohol, patients often need a well-controlled environment for a period of several months in the initial stages of their treatment. If the behavior disorder is sufficiently bizarre, as in delirium tremens or Korsakoff's syndrome, hospitalization is definitely indicated for the treatment of acute symptoms. Should the treatment of any alcoholic disorder stop with detoxification, however, the only accomplishment is a patient who is in better physical shape to continue drinking. Treatment must be oriented to personality rehabilitation. An environment in which the patient cannot secure alcohol and in which a full program of activities is available when the patient is ready is ideal.

Interpersonal relationships. Interpersonal relationships of a therapeutic nature are one of the alcoholic patient's greatest needs, and the establishment of such relationships is not easy. The major problems are the patient's inability to face his own problems and fears, his skillful rationalization and minimization of his drinking, his extreme sensitivity, his characteristic ambivalence, and his critically rebellious attitude toward hospitalization which develops in a month or two after his admission.

The patient usually comes for treatment in a poor physical condition after a period of prolonged drinking and is concerned about himself and anxious to be helped. He may be a little ashamed and sensitive about his drinking so that special care is indicated to keep from reinforcing such feelings about himself. As he improves physically, which occurs fairly quickly, he is grateful, congenial, and obviously enjoys feeling well physically again. It is here that personnel most often make the mistake of accepting the patient's explanations and reassurances at face value and letting the patient know that they expect much from him. The patient's minimizing of his difficulties and his rationalization of his behavior at this stage are clever camouflage. A neutral attitude of understanding without being overly sympathetic should be followed. No criticism or judgment, expressed or implied, should be indulged. The patient seems so rational that it is difficult to avoid the temptation to reason him out of his alcoholism. Although the patient will tell much, careful listening will indicate that there is also much that is not being told, and the latter is the more important of the two. The patient may brag about episodes which should be calmly listened to without comment. A direct approach to or comment on the patient's problems or drinking should be avoided because of the extreme sensitivity behind the patient's calm manner. As soon as possible the patient should be encouraged to participate in a daily program of activities, even though he may almost be able to convince the nurse that for him it is not necessary since he is quite well, has learned his lesson, and will be all right forever. Behind the patient's smooth facade is a lonely and fearful individual who is unable to look at his fears or admit his problems.

Physically well and usually coherent and impressive by comparison with his admission behavior, the patient then wants to go home. Any suggestion that he begin to come to grips with his problems brings forth the next difficulty in interpersonal relationships. The patient becomes rebellious and critical, turning on everyone associated with the institution. This behavior should be accepted without criticism or any disciplinary retaliation. The patient is now threatened. Anxiety makes its obvious appearance, and considerable resentment and hostility are expressed in words and negativism. This is a critical period for the patient, and interest in him should not be withdrawn. The hostility may be expressed, and its expression in the direction of personnel should be promoted. Once this phase begins to subside, improvement may be expected.

Most alcoholic patients are ambivalent in their emotional reactions to other people, and evidences of this are to be expected and calmly accepted. It is part and parcel of the patient's problems and is best expressed in the neutral atmosphere the patient needs.

Physical needs. Alcoholic patients need careful attention to complete physical rehabilitation. A diet high in vitamins and with an above average caloric intake helps in the initial stages to promote recovery. Attention should be paid to all phases of personal hygiene since most patients have neglected it thoroughly prior to admission. Not only should physical cleanliness be promoted, but also particular efforts should be directed to the cultivation of personal appearance for its psychologic aspect. As the patient's physical condition improves, he will need all his assets in the difficult period of readjustment.

As soon as possible the patient should be placed on a regular routine which emphasizes health habits, including exercise. Any defects or infections should receive prompt attention. Disfiguring scars that may have been acquired on a spree should be corrected if possible.

Protection. The patient's protective needs are related to the stage of his illness during hospitalization. When he is confused, disoriented, and restless, he may injure himself unintentionally and should therefore be constantly observed to prevent injury. As he recovers, if any depression is evident, the danger of suicide is present. The patient should be closely observed, kept active if possible, given an outlet for his hostility, and given the emotional support of personnel through interest and attention.

When the patient becomes rebellious, he needs observation to prevent an escape from the institution. He may also try to injure himself in an attempt to convince his family and hospital personnel that home is the best place for him.

Group relations. The alcoholic patient tends to be in but not of groups.

He will need tactful direction to participate, will need help in toning down his superior attitude toward those he thinks are sick, and will need encouragement to accept any responsibility for group activities. Any particular talent or ability the patient has should be promoted in group activities. Careful supervision to determine what patients, if any, are upset by the patient's comments during his critical period should be observed. When the patient's behavior is detrimental to others, free ventilation before personnel may help to tone him down with others. If the patient shows a tendency to associate with personnel and not with other patients, he may be brought into group activities through participation with personnel in the group.

Convalescence. The patient usually continues his rationalization, minimization, and anxiety into the convalescent period. These mechanisms should be identified for what they are in order to avoid supporting the patient on unsafe grounds. Evidences of real relationships with others or signs of real improvement should be promoted. Conversation or activities that indicate the patient's view of himself is becoming more realistic should also be recognized for the improvement they indicate, although no particular attention should be drawn to them because of the patient's sensitivity. If the patient is permitted out for visits and returns with the odor of alcohol, no great issue should be made of the episode before the patient, nor should criticism be voiced. It is a wise idea to expect little from the alcoholic patient in order to avoid being surprised by relapses or unexpected signs that the patient's adjustive ability is not as good as it seems on the surface. On the other hand, the patient should never be made aware of any such attitude.

References

McCarthy, Raymond G.: Alcoholism, American Journal of Nursing **59**:203-205, Feb. 1959.

Noyes, Arthur P., and Kolb, Lawrence C.: Modern Clinical Psychiatry, ed. 6, Philadelphia, 1963, W. B. Saunders Co., pp. 165-181.

Quiros, Alyce: Adjusting nursing techniques to the treatment of alcoholic patients, Nursing Outlook **5**:276-279, May 1957.

Sorenson, K. and Fagen, R.: The hospitalized skid row alcoholic, Nursing Forum **2**:48, 1963.

Thompson, George N.: Acute and chronic alcoholic conditions. In Arieti, Silvana, editor: American handbook of psychiatry, New York, 1959, Basic Books, Inc., vol. 2, pp. 1203-1221.

Chapter XXI

Nursing care of patients
who depend on drugs

D rugs, like alcohol, offer emotionally unstable persons a prop to aid them through the crises and the give-and-take of existence. Because of the definite effect on the organism, certain drugs offer the compensatory effects of making reality seem more pleasant and the individual feel more capable of dealing with it. Although the effects of the drugs will account for their use by a person with susceptible personality, what makes that personality need their support is again a question without a specific answer. The etiologic factors of most significance are to be found in the personality structure of the individual. Morphine, cocaine, marihuana, and the barbiturates are popular among persons who habitually depend upon drugs as an aid to adjustment.

Opium and its derivatives have long been used by mankind for the purpose of producing an euphoric sense of well-being and tranquility. The most commonly used is heroin. Having been exposed to the comforting effects of the drug, unstable persons resort again and again to it under stress and pressure until the habit is firmly established. Opium alkaloids produce both physical and psychologic dependence. In other words, their continued use so affects metabolism that the individual finds it difficult to function without their use. Thus the patient's efforts to help himself become doubly difficult. The initiation of the habit is commonly blamed on physicians, and although there are probably a number of instances in which the first experience with the effects of morphine came under a physician's care, it is open to serious doubt as to whether the majority of instances of addiction began thus. The acquisition of morphine addiction is related to the opportunity to acquire the drug, as well as to the need for it, and it is questionable to say the least that reputable physicians make it a habit to continue furnishing a patient with sufficient quantities of any opium derivatives to encourage addiction. The habit is more likely to be developed through association with other addicts with whom a source of supply for the drug is established. That opportunity to obtain morphine is a factor is illustrated by the fact that addiction among members of the medical and allied professions is more common than in the general population. The medical group have ready access to the drug.

The prolonged use of morphine tends to result in social isolation and deterioration of personal habits. The patient's physical dependence upon the drug and his inability to tolerate the anxiety and physical symptoms that go with a lack of morphine drive him to almost any lengths to secure it. Because of this and because the Harrison Act makes the possession and use of the opium derivatives without a license a criminal offense, the morphine addict often comes into conflict with the law. The patient becomes increasingly less efficient and devotes less energy to ordinary goals and ambitions. His life becomes increasingly oriented to securing an adequate supply of his drug, and the amount needed tends to increase gradually as the body builds a tolerance. Many addicts take in a single dose a sufficient amount of morphine to kill a person not accustomed to the drug. The physical picture of the patient is rather typical: emaciation, grayish complexion, tremors, constricted pupils, poor speech coordination, coated tongue, halitosis, and marked constipation.

The abrupt withdrawal of morphine or other opium alkaloids produces a definite withdrawal or abstinence syndrome. The severity of the symptoms will depend upon the length of time the patient has been an addict and the dosage to which he is accustomed. Initial symptoms are yawning, lacrimation, sneezing, perspiration, and restlessness which are followed by anorexia, muscular pains, and tremors. More severe manifestations are fever, increased restlessness and irritability, insomnia, and elevated blood pressure. Vomiting, diarrhea, weight loss, and prostration mark the most severe reactions. Because of the dangers of the withdrawal reaction, the sudden and complete removal of narcotics has been possible only since the use of the tranquilizing drugs has given evidence of the ability to control the symptoms of withdrawal. Initial reports reveal that chlorpromazine, for example, has effectively alleviated the withdrawal symptoms in narcotic addiction and has made it possible for patients to participate more easily in psychotherapy.

In addition to opium and its derivatives, Demerol Sodium and methadon are narcotics that produce physical dependency, and the abrupt withdrawal of either can cause an abstinence syndrome. Methadon can however be used as a substitute for morphine in the process of withdrawal because its abstinence syndrome is less severe than the one in morphinism.

Cocaine and its derivatives are resorted to by susceptible persons for the feeling of well-being they induce. However, cocaine addiction is not as common as other forms. The drug may be taken by hypodermic injection or by sniffing the powdered form of cocaine through the nostrils. Patients under the influence of these drugs experience a sense of euphoria accompanied by motor restlessness. Prolonged use results in habit deterioration, a dulling of the ethical or moral judgment, confusion, and somatic delusions. The expression "cocaine bug" derives from a rather common somatic delusion of worms or bugs crawling under the skin. Physical symptoms include dilated pupils, rapid pulse, weakness, and emaciation. The withdrawal of cocaine is not accompanied by a definite syndrome since the drug does not induce physical dependency.

Marihuana is derived from the flowering tops of the hemp plant which grows extensively throughout the United States. The actual extent of its use is unknown, but it is presumed to be on the increase since it is so easily obtained. The usual method of administration is by smoking cigarettes, called reefers, which are made of the dried leaves of the plant. Patients first become apprehensive and fearful and then euphoric. They experience a sense of unrealness and disturbance in time sensation, for time seems to pass very slowly. Hallucinatory experiences may occur, as well as restless excitement. After several hours the patient becomes sleepy, and after awakening he has none of the usual hang-over that goes with the use of alcohol or other drugs. The withdrawal of marihuana is not accompanied by physiologic symptoms.

The use of barbiturates has become a major social problem because of their extensive prescription by the medical profession, their calming effect, and the ease with which they can be obtained. The various preparations are widely used for their quieting effect and to produce sleep. Patients with neurotic tendencies find them a comfortable prop to allay anxiety and apprehension. Various preparations, such as Nembutal, Seconal, Luminal, and Sodium Amytal are taken consistently over a long period of time. Overdoses within a short period can cause a typical acute toxic reaction with delirium or death. Prolonged use may cause dullness and lethargy, and if continued for years, it may also produce gradual personality deterioration accompanied by organic symptoms such as memory defect, confusion, disorientation, poor judgment, and reduced intellectual capacity. This, however, is not the inevitable outcome since some persons use barbiturates for years without personality or intellectual deterioration. In a person accustomed to a steady dosage, the withdrawal of the drug abruptly may precipitate convulsions. In any case the anxiety and tension that have been controlled by the barbiturates become evident, and the patient is usually quite uncomfortable. The reliance upon barbiturates is rather extensive among groups of people who are familiar with their effect. The nurse who takes Benzedrine to stay awake on night duty and barbiturates to sleep during the day is not so rare as one might wish.

The treatment of drug addiction is based on the withdrawal of the drug, physical rehabilitation, and then the more difficult step of personality rehabilitation. In drugs that result in physical dependency, the first problem is to reduce that dependency, which is accomplished either by gradual withdrawal of the drug or by immediate withdrawal and administration of tranquilizing drugs. If gradual withdrawal is used, the patient is given 15 mg. or ¼ grain of morphine every four or six hours, usually the latter, and the dose is gradually reduced over a period of days until the patient receives no more. The length of time involved and the particular method of reducing the dosage may vary in different institutions. The patient will experience some discomfort with this type of withdrawal, but the reaction will not be nearly so severe as if abrupt withdrawal were practiced. With drugs that do not produce physical dependency, abrupt withdrawal is the treatment of choice. Small doses of sedatives or chemotherapy may be used to help control restlessness and anxiety. Fluids must be forced, and the diet should be high in vitamins and calories, with vitamin supplements if necessary. In the treatment of drug addiction generally, the patient must be in a controlled environment for a sufficiently long period to enable the habit of living without the drug to be established. As in the treatment of alcoholism, to discharge the patient when he reaches a good physical level simply sends him home in better condition to return to his reliance on drugs. Psychotherapy is directed toward helping the patient reach the source of his problems and toward developing better techniques for solving emotional problems than the use of drugs to control his anxiety. Some of the pessimism of the medical profession toward the treatment of alcoholism is repeated in the attitude toward the rehabilitation of drug addicts.

Nursing care

The nursing care of patients suffering from drug addiction requires a high degree of alertness, tact, and real skill in the ability to differentiate true symptoms from pseudosymptoms. To outwit the patient's efforts to circumvent the removal of dependence upon drugs while at the same time meeting his emotional needs requires a diplomat of the first order.

Psychotherapeutic environment. The essence of a psychotherapeutic environment for patients with this type of behavior disorder centers around control. The surroundings should prevent the accessibility of the drug so completely that it is possible to be tactful about the prohibition and should make it difficult for the patient to leave on impulse. Facilities for the treatment of acute episodes, such as the withdrawal syndrome in morphinism or the acute toxic reaction in barbital poisoning, should be readily available. The atmosphere should be pleasant and cheerful and not too stimulating. Trained personnel with an understanding of the patient's illness are an absolute necessity.

Interpersonal relationships. Patients who develop a psychologic dependence upon drugs are inadequate persons who, if they ever knew how, have unlearned any toleration for anxiety and frustration. They need relationships that contribute to their self-confidence and self-respect, that satisfy their emotional needs sufficiently to promote a feeling of comfort, and that make socialization worth while. Particular problems center around evasion, negativism, hostility, dependence, and malingering. A relatively permissive atmosphere with a strain of firmness is indicated.

Evasion and escape from responsibility are rather typical, as would be expected. It is important to identify this mechanism and to accept it matter-of-factly while holding the patient to certain minimum standards, such as group participation, care of personal hygiene, and adequate diet intake. The patient may have to clean his teeth, but the fact that he does not want to can be accepted and not ignored or pushed aside. To accept behavior without sanctioning it is the principle to be followed. Negativism and hostility can be matter-of-factly faced, and the avoidance of any open issue over authority is helpful. Very thorough orientation of the patient in the initial stages of hospitalization is an effective preventive measure so that the patient knows in advance what is expected of him.

Efficiency and positiveness on the part of the nurse do much to promote a sense of confidence and security in the patient and constitute a good background on which to build relationships. Hesitancy and uncertainty may be exploited by the patient, especially in evasion and malingering. Dependency of the patient on the nurse should not be rewarded with approval or favoritism, however.

A great deal of tact is required in observing and interpreting the patient's physical symptoms. The addict is prone to exaggerate and pretend in order to secure medication over and beyond his real need and is utterly amoral in this respect. Study of the patient and assessment of his actual physical condition required good judgment and are developed through practice. If this particular form of behavior is to be handled well, it is necessary to maintain a very neutral reaction when the behavior occurs. It is one of the major pitfalls in relationships since failure to deceive the nurse may call forth hostility and deception of the nurse may call forth a lack of confidence which the patient really needs. Alertness to the psychologic significance of the personal relationships involved helps to reduce the possibility of retaliatory measures against the patient. The patient needs at all times acceptance, friendliness, and security.

If the patient is receiving experimental drugs, very careful observation and recording of all aspects of patient behavior and physical condition are extremely important.

Physical needs. The physical needs of the patient are related to the stage and degree of illness. Following an overdose of a barbiturate, a stuporous patient needs the same care that any unconscious patient requires, with special attention to respiratory difficulties associated with increased secretion of mucus and depression of the respiratory center that are reflections of the nature of the barbiturates. With a delirium or the withdrawal syndrome of morphine addiction, personal hygiene and good skin care are important aspects of nursing care. Frequent massage and protection against skin friction are helpful. Fluids are forced, and as soon as nausea has been controlled, an adequate diet through frequent small feedings should be encouraged. The process of graduation to a regular diet is promoted.

Accurate observation and evaluation of physical symptoms are important to the patient because of the relationship between his physical dependence or intoxication to the symptoms he shows. His needs in regard to treatment will be determined on the basis of reports of such observations.

Attention to personal hygiene, including every aspect of personal cleanliness and the establishment of a health routine, is usually necessary since the majority of patients have been careless in this respect for many years. Patients who are addicted to drugs tend to be rather disinterested in keeping themselves and their environment reasonably clean and neat, and the initial establishment of habits needs constant reinforcement until the patient learns to accept the responsibility.

Protective needs. A protective atmosphere is imperative in the care of a patient who is pathologically dependent upon drugs. Protective needs fall into three categories: prevention of access to the drug of choice or any substitute, protection against injury during an acute episode, and protection against self-injury.

When he is admitted, the patient and his personal effects should be thoroughly searched, and personal effects should be removed until any possible source of drugs is eliminated. Visitors and communications should be subject to some form of control to prevent smuggling. Many trusting relatives and, unfortunately, some overly sympathetic personnel may be so misguided as to feel that they are doing the patient a favor by supplying him with drugs. Another particular source of danger is persons close to the patient who have a masked hostility toward him. Not understanding their own motivation, such persons may well contribute to the patient's difficulties by furnishing him with contraband.

Drugs in the hospital should be kept under strict control, and medication given should be taken under supervision at the time of administration to prevent hoarding. The patient's actual symptoms should be carefully evaluated to prevent unnecessary medication.

The patient may injure himself at any stage of his illness in an attempt to gain sympathy or to force the use of medication for the relief of pain. The danger is that the patient may injure himself more seriously than he intends. Emotional support, a program of activities that keeps the patient busy, and close observation are preventive measures. If depression or despondency is present, precautions against suicide should be taken.

To prevent injury during an acute episode, the patient should be closely observed, and protective measures such as the use of sideboards should be taken when necessary.

Group relations. Socialization on a satisfactory level is one of the ultimate aims in the treatment plan for patients with a dependency on drugs. Therefore, as early as possible the patient should be introduced to group activities on a planned basis. Every asset or resource the patient has should be exploited to use group relationships to contribute to his self-confidence. Being among patients who have similar problems is a help in itself since it reduces the patient's sense of loneliness and isolation. Shared fears and difficulties are easier to face than fears that are kept to one's self. Ventilation and emotional catharsis in the group may be permitted, provided that they do not produce marked anxiety. Again it should be remembered that patients are more tolerant of each other than personnel are likely to realize and that sensitivity to how the patient feels is the important criterion, rather than how personnel feel. In any instance, group interaction should be encouraged, and the patient should not be permitted to isolate himself.

Convalescence. The patient's hospitalization should be prolonged from four to six months at least, and the convalescent period is usually a difficult one. A regular routine that gives the patient a balance of work and play should be established and carried through. During this period strict attention should be paid to the establishment of habits, and the tendency of the patient to evade should be faced and overcome. The value of convalescence lies in the patient's opportunity to meet situations and routine without evasion and to learn for himself that he can get along without dependence on outside help. Responsibility for himself and the care of his own immediate environment should be promoted. If the patient begins to develop insight, its beginning stages are likely to be accompanied by an exacerbation of anxiety. Reassurance through personal interest and encouragement is then necessary. If the patient is to remain free of his previous addiction, the convalescent period must contribute to his sense of importance and his confidence in his ability to meet problems of his own.

References

LaLancette, T.: The nurse and the narcotic addict, Journal of Psychiatric Nursing 1:29, Jan. 1963.

Noyes, Arthur P., and Kolb, Lawrence C.: Modern clinical psychiatry, ed. 6, Philadelphia, 1963, W. B. Saunders Co., pp. 473-481.

Nyswander, Marie: Drug addictions. In Arieti, Silvana, editor: American handbook of psychiatry, New York, 1959, Basic Books, Inc., vol. 1, pp. 614-622.

Children: Their behavior and problems

Chapter XXii

Developmental problems of children

I t is fitting that this chapter on child psychiatry appear here, sequentially. The focus on children and their problems evolved out of the study of adults, their behavior and mental illnesses. At this point we are well aware of the significance of childhood experiences to the adult personality (see Chapters III and IV). Biographical data, from birth to the onset of an emotional illness, are important to the understanding of the underlying factors which contribute to an individual's makeup.

Historic review

Although evidence is available that peoples of ancient times and numerous cultures had concern for children and their welfare, no period in history has contributed so much to the understanding of children as has the twentieth century. Therefore, it is not strange that many refer to it as "the century of the child."

In the past, the role of the child was to obey, to serve, to honor, and to conform to his parents. His individuality and personal feelings were suppressed lest he be considered a bad child. The will of the parents or guardians dominated the child's life. Rigid religious codes often determined the morality of right and wrong. Children were loved but were needed more. From a very early age, children were given specific chores which were essential to the vitality of family life.

During the eighteenth and nineteenth centuries several writers of literature drew attention to the natural development of children, their problems, and their pedagogy. Jean Jacques Rousseau's *Emile* and Charles Dickens' numerous volumes, *Oliver Twist* in particular, are examples of books in which men brought before the public the conditions that surrounded children at these times. Some men began to look at children as individuals. Pestalozzi (1774) observed and recorded the behavior of his young son and emphasized the individuality of children as human beings. Similarly, Tiedemann in 1787 published the observations of the total growth and development of his children. In 1877, Darwin described the forces of human survival as evident in child development. Preyer's work on the mind of the child is said to have been the beginning of child psychology. There were many others who contributed to the interest and study of children during these centuries and thus set the stage for further progress in the twentieth century.

In the first half of the twentieth century, tremendous progress was made in the study of the child and his problems. Several forces were at work concomitantly which created this impetus. First, the scientific method had become an established method of enlightenment and had permeated the realms of medicine and the social sciences. The social sciences were accepted as respectable areas of knowledge within our institutions of higher learning and were acknowledged for their professional value. Pedagogy, education curriculums, and methods were examined and questioned. Theories on child rearing were shaken.

Alfred Binet made a break-through when he published his famous scale of measuring intelligence in relation to mental age in 1905. The Binet-Simon scale demonstrated an important individual difference among children and stimulated the serious examination of human intelligence and the learning processes. Terman adopted this scale for use with American children and initiated much activity in further scientific study. Arnold Gesell and his associates contributed greatly to the objective observation and study of children through the use of modern and scientific techniques. John Dewey, philosopher and psychologist, introduced his revolutionary theories on child rearing and education by declaring the need for children "to learn by doing." Unfortunately in the implementation of his theories some of his enthusiastic but less knowledgeable followers created abuses rather than uses for his theories.

Psychiatry and pediatrics witnessed many important changes in their knowledge and practice. In pediatrics, medical care became a planned routine for young children and preventive care became a household concern. Dynamic psychiatry recognized the need to understand the whole person—his early experiences and his life's experiences, as well as his symptoms. These are the threads which lead to the origins of mental illness. A biographic history is now an essential component of the patient's personal data. It has become self-evident that childhood maladjustments require the attention and therapeutic skills of psychiatrists and psychologists.

The law and courts also showed concern for the treatment of delinquent children during this period. Prior to 1899, the law made no distinction between a child and an adult offender. In the early 1900's, juvenile courts and the probationary ruling were established. This provided the means whereby youngsters in trouble could be examined by psychiatrists and psychologists.

All of these factors and others were culminating toward a clearer understanding of youngsters as individuals, their behavior, and the underlying motives for their problems. It wasn't until 1922 that the "demonstration child guidance clinics" were first established. These clinics provided the services of a therapeutic team composed of a psychiatrist, a psychologist, and a social worker who dealt with the "problem" children referred by schools, child-caring agencies, parents, and others. The value of these clinics became widely known, and by 1930 there were about 500 throughout the continent. The child guidance clinics demonstrated their therapeutic effectiveness with children and incorporated the concept of "attitude therapy" involving parents and teachers. This led to more careful examination and analysis of the family and school situations as influences on childhood behavior problems.

Psychiatrists continued to seek the meaning behind behavior symptoms for both adults and children. However, children were cryptic and enigmatic for the adult not living in a child's world. Anna Freud conceived the theory that children seek self-expression through play. Not only was this a means of providing an acceptable method for the child to express hostility, anxiety, and insecurity, but it also afforded the child a therapeutic emotional release.

Today child psychiatry is accepted as a special and important field of psychiatry to be included in medical education, nursing education, and teacher education. Child psychiatrists are partners with pediatricians in the care of children in hospitals and clinics. Schools, juvenile courts, nurses, teachers, lawyers, and other institutions and individuals involved with children are more cognizant of the resources available to help youngsters with disturbing behavior. And most important, the public and the parents and guardians of children are being educated with respect to children's behavior problems and the various means available to help them to help their youngsters.

Childhood and parenthood

Leo Kanner has stated: "Childhood is a collective term. It includes all ages between the neonatal period and the termination of puberty. It carries the individual from a condition of complete biologic helplessness to the threshold of self-dependence and creative activity."* And at the end of this period, "socialization" is the major achievement. Childhood is a part of the continuum of life for the individual. Socialization, as a developmental process, is used by Kanner to identify three periods of childhood. The first, the period of elementary socialization, spans the first 15 to 18 months of life accompanied by total dependence upon and interaction with his parents and other individuals within his immediate environment. From about 18 months to 5 years the second, the period of domestic socialization, evolves. This is the time when the child learns about himself and his environment in relation to his family. Simple conversational skills and elementary understanding of numbers are gained. Recognition of authority and obedience to orders are developed. Habit training is a

---

*From Kanner, Leo: Child psychiatry, Springfield, Ill., 1962, Charles C Thomas, Publisher, p. 33.

major activity and helps the child to become a greater part of the family and to progress toward greater socialization beyond the family.

Within this period, investigators have studied patterns of behavior identified as resistance to dependence on and direction from adults. Annoying as this behavior may be to parents and other adults, most authors agree that it is a healthy aspect of childhood, illustrative of the child's desire for self-dependence and personality growth. This negativism is therefore to be treated as a phase of personality development and with the same understanding as physical growth. Understanding and accepting this type of behavior matter-of-factly, without hostility and vengence, will go far in avoiding a child-parent emotional blow up and a contest of wills. The frequent verbal expressions of negativism if casually ignored will do more good than harm. The daily routine may be consistently enforced with the accompaniment of affection and security in the parent-child relationship. This resistance behavior is most often seen between the ages of 2 to 4 years and is of varying duration in each child.

The third phase, the period of communal socialization, brings the child out and into greater involvement with the community, its people and agencies. His activities are less within the home and more with the school, the team, the church, the gang, the club, and the neighbors. His world enlarges as do his experiences in preparation for an ever-expanding world. He learns the give-and-take of responsibilities and the significance of mutual respect. Physically and intellectually his growth has reached its peak at about the sixteenth year.

A wise man once said, "Give me a child for the first seven years and I will give you a man." Another remark often heard is the following, "He is just like his father or his mother." These are two common sayings which make obvious the penetrating influence exerted by parents and other adults in the immediate environment of the child. Many say that claim of parental resemblance is physiognomy; however, as one looks more carefully, it is the behavior, the mannerisms, the preferences, and the dislikes which distinguish a child of particular parents or a specific family.

From the time of his conception to his birth and throughout his childhood the attitudes of the parents condition the personality of the child and compose the fibers for his self-image. Was he wanted or was his conception an accident? Did his birth present physical and/or emotional problems for the parents? Was his arrival into the family a burdensome responsibility? Affirmative or negative responses to these and other related questions may not be readily expressed by parents but they are reflected in their attitudes toward their children. Oftentimes, the subtlety of the expression of an attitude escapes the observer but not the victim. The study of a child and his problems, therefore, must of necessity include an examination and an understanding of both the child and his parents, if a wholistic approach is to be achieved. Attitudes, positive or negative, are born of relationships and experiences in an individual's life and his sensitive response to these. This fact applies to parents' attitudes as well as to those of children and should be kept in mind when considering a wholistic approach. Total love without dislike, total acceptance without some rejection, is a rare thing in our society, but the predominance of one feeling or the other becomes obvious in relationships with children.

The love of parents for their children is manifested in many ways and results in the acceptance of each child for his own sake. The presence of this wholesome attitude permeates most, if not all, aspects of the family's vitality and is inescapable to the observer. What creates this attitude? Many have sought the answer, but few have learned the secret. It is to be found in the substance of the parents and individuals making up the family, their parents, and the parents who preceded them. The evolutionary relationship and influence of parents on children may touch each successive generation.

Similarly, the dislike of parents for a child or children, whether on a conscious or an unconscious level, is displayed in the multiple forms rejection can take. A parent's rejection of a child may stem from many motives—some obvious and some rather obscure. Growth in social maturity and adult responsibility is an important factor in an individual's attitudes toward marriage and family. The meaning of mothering an infant is directly related to the mother's concept of herself as a person, a wife, and a mother. An illegitimate child is often rejected for personal, societal, and economic reasons. How the parents view the purpose of the child in their husband-wife relationship is significant. A child may be conceived for purposes of holding a husband, keeping a wife busy, curing an emotional problem, maturing the husband and/or wife, and obtaining an heir. If the infant's birth, for some reason or another, does not fulfill the anticipated purpose, the resulting hatred, hostility, and guilt are manifested in overt and covert rejection.

Kanner distinguishes three principal forms of rejecting behavior. The first is overt hostility and neglect. Obvious maltreatment of the infant or child through neglect, verbal and/or physical abuse, deprivation of clothing or food, annoyance, scolding, ridicule, and harsh punishment may be imposed. The absence of holding and fondling the infant, the purposeful delegation by the parents of the infant to another adult, and the mother's immediate return to work regardless of need are a few of the subtle socially acceptable ways of rejecting. Such a child grows with a craving for affection and lacks the ability of deep emotional response.

The second form of rejection cited is perfectionism, wherein the mother, in attempting to fulfill the mother-role society extols, camouflages her rejection by projecting an imperfection on the child whom she will traumatize in her efforts to make him perfect. Paternal rejection may also be expressed in making the "perfect all-around boy." Needless to say, this creates in the child a feeling of dissatisfaction with himself. He works and strives constantly toward the lofty standards and expectations set down by his parents, and when he doesn't succeed, he feels guilty, insecure, defeated, and hopeless.

Compensatory overprotection is the third form. Behavior manifesting overprotection is not always motivated by rejection. A mother whose previous experience has deprived her of another child may fear the loss of this new precious child, and so she becomes overprotective. The mother, motivated by underlying rejection, uses the overprotective behavior as a means of maintaining a conscious image of being a good mother and thus keeps her rejection down in her unconscious.

A mother's overprotection of a child, regardless of its cause, may result in either a spoiled brat who dominates the parents and household, or a child smothered by love who becomes greatly dependent on and dominated by his mother. Thus his maturation and emancipation are inhibited.

Nurses and attitudes

Nurses have numerous opportunities to observe the attitudes of children and parents. Their encounters are many in their roles as nurses in homes, in schools, in pediatricians' offices, in clinics, and in hospitals. As a member of the community, she has friendships with the neighborhood youngsters, and the Sunday school class. However a great deal is missed or lost unless nurses are perceptive, and unless they are equipped with a fine antenna to pick up and identify attitudes subtly expressed or camouflaged. Observed behavior, verbal and nonverbal, needs to be seen for its true meaning. The moment's scene is related to what went on before and what is yet to follow, if one is to understand the drama completely. The hero and the villain are defined as they act with the other members of the group. The characters and the setting are important to the meaning.

In addition to observing, the nurse in the clinical situation must report accurately. An anecdotal account should be written, and where necessary, the nurse's reaction or interpretation may be included, clearly identified as such. Let us not forget that nurses are human and react to people and situations. But their education has taught them to be aware of their reacting and reactions. They need to develop the ability to know, to define, and to accept their reactions. When there is confusion or great emotional involvement, the nurse has resources she may turn to for assistance, such as psychiatric nurses, supervisors, psychiatrists, and psychologists. Self-understanding is essential to helping others.

The nurse whose position brings her into close contact with children would benefit by deliberating several questions. How does she feel about children? Why does she feel this way? Does she like or dislike children? What is her usual behavior as a nurse with them? What major purpose does she serve as a nurse with children? How does she feel about the various types of parents she encounters? Does she tend to blame them or accept them in their roles?

As nurses are human, so are parents. Some parents' attitudes toward their children may be very disturbing and arouse much anger and hostility in the nurse. Coupled with the child's behavior toward the parents, the nurse may very easily judge and blame the parents for the child's problems. This judgment is inescapably reflected in her treatment of the parents and child and renders her ineffectual in helping either party. Usually both the parents and child need help. It is important to assess this fact and to recognize that the parents' behavior is often an expression of their problems which require understanding and therapy.

Age and behavior

The changes between infancy and puberty occur imperceptibly and gradually. Yet, they are as distinct as the diaper and the long trousers! Typical behavior patterns are identified as specific to each stage of childhood and serve as a means of identifying one aspect of social maturation. Unfortunately this typical behavior is used by parents and professionals as a rigid yardstick rather than as a flexible one. Children tend to express their problems in behavior appropriate for their age group. Leo Kanner has stated:

"Resentment and frustration find expression in infants through breath holding spells, which reach their peak toward the end of the second year, are reduced in frequency about one third in the third year, and have all but disappeared by the end of the fourth year. Their place is taken by temper tantrums, which arise from the same type of situation which at an earlier age had precipitated the breath holding spells. Temper tantrums, in turn, sporadic at 2 years, become more frequent at 3, are maintained at a fairly even rate until 9, and peter out at around 11 to 12 years. They are displaced by sullenness and argumentation; the tantrums themselves are of a different caliber at 9 to 10 than they are at 3 to 4; the older child does not throw himself on the floor or bang his head in rage."[*]

It is important to keep in mind that the recognition of a behavior problem is also conditioned by the mother's evaluation and feeling about the child and his readiness for habit training, socialization, and responsibility. One mother may show great concern about bed wetting in a one year old, whereas another may recognize the problem only when the seven year old is being prepared for camp. Regressive behavior manifested by a six year old's request for breast feeding may be an expression of his inability to cope with his craving for his mother's love in any other way.

---

[*]From Kanner, Leo: Child psychiatry, Springfield, Ill., 1962, Charles C Thomas, Publisher, p. 45.

References

Christina, Sr. Mary: The role of the nurse in child caring institutions, Journal of Psychiatric Nursing 2:281-285, May-June, 1964.

Crutcher, R.: Child psychiatry; A history of its development, Journal of Biological and Pathological Interpersonal Relations 6:191-201, June, 1943.

Hillsman, Gladys M.: Now I am a person, Nursing Outlook 11:172-179, Mar. 1963.

Kanner, Leo: Child psychiatry, Springfield, Ill., 1962, Charles C Thomas, Publisher, pp. 1-72.

Lewis, Richard S.: The other child, New York, 1951, Grune & Stratton, Inc.

Noyes, Arthur P. and Kolb, Lawrence C.: Modern clinical psychiatry, ed. 6, Philadelphia, 1963, W. B. Saunders Co., pp. 482-499.

Chapter XXiii

Nursing care of children with functionally based behavior problems

Although the underlying dynamics of mental disorders in children are closely allied to those of adults, a child's behavior must be analyzed and evaluated in light of his development. This task is difficult and depends on the child's communication skills, imagination, and cooperation. A child's problems are manifested in behavior which causes disruptions in the routine of his daily living, in his relationships with his parents and family, and sometimes in the affairs of the community. The disturbance created by the child is his way of saying he has deep, personal discord and will someone please help. The behavior is a sign, a symptom, and not an ugly nature, an inherited tendency, or a weakness. During childhood, as pointed out earlier, numerous, rapid changes take place which are often accompanied by normal problems. These normal problems are associated with the activities of daily living.

Feeding-eating problems

The feeding problem is the mother's; the eating problem is the child's. It is often difficult to distinguish which originated the situation. The mother's problem may be related to her desire to give the best care to her infant and child and to the anxiety which results from her attempts. Time schedules and specified foods and the maximum amounts of each, rigidly applied, are causes to stir even a young infant to rebellion. As the infant or child expresses his objection to the feeding routine, the mother becomes more convinced that the child has a problem and tries harder, and then anxiety and tension increase. Several experiments with infants and children have been carried out which demonstrate the child's ability to select satisfactorily his nourishment in the kind and amounts to meet his optimal needs.

In the absence of a physical illness as the cause of anorexia, psychologic disturbances are usually the contributing factors. Some frequent clues may be the child's preference for specific foods only, his refusal of food at mealtime but not in-between feedings, and his refusal of food from the mother or father and acceptance of food from other sources. Or, the child may refuse all food. The cause for loss of appetite should be examined from the point of view of the child and the end he hopes to achieve by his behavior, from the point of view of the mother or other adult who feeds the child (their relationship to the child and their attitude toward his feeding), and, last, from the point of view of the feeding technique.

The child's refusal of food may be his method of gaining the fondling, cuddling, and attention of an otherwise unaffectionate mother who feeds and cares for him automatically. He may have learned that his negativism gives him control over the household and permits him to have his way. He may be expressing his unhappiness or depression. The parent-child relationship is basic to all considerations. The mother's method of feeding the child could be controlled by underlying feelings, such as rejection, overprotection, anxiety, lack of knowledge, adherence to a set routine, confusion, and fear.

The treatment of children with feeding-eating disorders must obviously involve the child, his symptoms, and his parents. Very often, anxiety over the child's malnourished condition prescribes symptomatic treatment, and the underlying causes are overlooked. Therefore, the symptoms may recur frequently. Mothers need guidance in dealing with the problem and are often advised to ignore the symptoms. Their anxiety and oversolicitude may prevent this approach from being successful. Between-meal feedings are discouraged, and the child's favorite foods are offered at mealtime as a means of interesting the child in eating. Small portions are recommended until he requests more. When the eating habit is reestablished, other foods may be introduced gradually. Concomitant with the direct attention to the problem is study of the child's underlying motivation. The mother is helped to understand her feelings and the contribution that she makes to the problem.

Anorexia nervosa is a general term used to designate severe loss of appetite and self-denial of food. This condition occurs more often in adolescents than in younger children and suggests a serious emotional disorder. The self-imposed starvation may jeopardize the child's life. Hospitalization and treatment in a controlled setting are recommended.

Another eating disorder is excessive eating. The reasons for overeating are related to some of the causes discussed previously. The oversolicitude of a well-intentioned mother may establish the habit of excessive eating. It may well be the best way a child has of gaining approval and expressions of affection from his parents. He may use large amounts of food to compensate for unsatisfied desires and frustrations. Treatment involves the child and his parents, his symptoms, and his purpose for eating as he does. For the adolescent obesity may be a problem of great magnitude because our society places considerable emphasis and significance on the "body beautiful." The parents view the situation as a serious handicap since it affects the child's social relationships and activities among his peers and in the community.

Pica designates a disorder that is characterized by the ingestion of substances having no nutritional value. The reasons for this condition are not fully understood. An infant often places toys and other objects (including the bedrails) in his mouth. Often the ingestion of paint causes serious lead poisoning. Bugs, worms, dirt, pebbles, strings, hair, buttons, and paper are some other objects which children may ingest habitually, which result in a variety of disorders. Preventive measures are indicated when this condition is first observed.

The nursing care of children with undereating and overeating disorders involves the observation of the child's behavior, and reocrds of the behavior are kept as a means of identifying the underlying causes. The nurse's warmth, interest, and affection for the child will go far in gaining his trust and perhaps cooperation in his therapy. The child's projection of his maternal attitudes to the nurse should be recognized and handled matter-of-factly, without retaliation and hostility. Keeping the child occupied, particularly an older child, will help to distract his attention and conversation from his symptoms. Patience and understanding are essential in the management of these patients.

Sleep disturbances

Sleep patterns of normal children show some variations, but when a child is disturbed, sleep behavior becomes a problem which is manifest in a wide range of symptoms from mild restlessness to wakefulness, insomnia, and excessive drowsiness and variations of these. When no physical disorder is present, emotional factors must be carefully examined. A brief period of psychotherapy may be indicated since sleep disturbances very often accompany other conditions such as anxiety, jealousy, insecurity, and psychoneurosis.

Problems of speech

The complex function of speech requires the use and synchronization of certain areas of the brain, the organs of vocalization and hearing, the intelligence and comprehension, and the emotional components involved in understanding and responsiveness. An impairment or disturbance in speech may denote trouble in any of these areas. When the speech disorder has no organic basis, the cause is usually associated with the child's parental and family situation and his emotional maladjustment. Delayed speech, prolonged baby talk, lisping, and stuttering are conditions which have strong emotional implications. Present-day studies tend to support the theory of their psychic origin.

Stuttering is the involuntary hesitation, the repetition of words, or the prolongation of sounds in speech. The frustration of the stutterer frequently causes him to go through certain body movements. Tossing of the head, facial grimaces, swallowing, gasping, clenching of the fists, jerking arm motions, and stamping of the feet are frequent when the child attempts to control or relieve his stuttering. Although it is recognized that stuttering indicates some underlying emotional disturbance, the manifestations of this behavior contributes additional difficulty to the development of his personality. A child who stutters becomes sensitive and self-conscious and shies away from social activities. Ridicule from children and insensitive adults causes him to withdraw and become seclusive—all of which, of course, contributes more to the child's tension and stuttering. Treatment should begin as soon as the stuttering becomes acute. If the child can be helped to resolve his emotional disorder early, his stuttering habit can then be relieved and further emotional trauma can be avoided. As the therapist works with the child and recognizes the dynamics of his problem, the parental relationship is also explored. The understanding and support of the parents and family in this complex problem are paramount. Speech therapy is an adjunct to psychotherapy and gives the child moral support. He is taught how to overcome his speech difficulties by relaxation and conscious control of his speech pattern. The method and the personal approach of the speech therapist, the nurses, and other personnel help the child regain his self-confidence and determination to work at overcoming his disorder.

Mutism is the inability to speak and is associated with other complex disorders such as childhood schizophrenia, early infantile autism, and hysteria. Nonverbal communication is a challenge to the nurse and requires her alert attention, her imaginativeness, her understanding of the child, and her sympathetic patience. Care of the child should not be an automatic routine in which things are done to him but should provide an opportunity for the child to participate to the degree that he is able. Direct questions should not dominate the conversation; rather, inflections in sentences should convey the invitation for the child to respond.

Problems in juvenile delinquency

Children whose actions and behavior violate the law frequently come to the attention of the courts. These children are classified juvenile delinquents. At the present time, the rate of juvenile delinquency is shamefully high. Although many persons have studied this problem, little understanding as to how delinquent children may be helped and rehabilitated has been achieved. The reasons for the troublesome behavior are closely allied to the feelings and needs of a child.

The range of delinquent behavior is very broad and includes minor misdemeanors, stealing, sexual acts, destruction of property, cruelty and injury to persons, drug addiction, and murder, to name a few. The motives causing such crimes are inherent in the child's personality and background. The responsibility and contribution of the parents and family to the child's problem are inescapable and are demonstrable in most cases.

Although the courts attempt to help children in trouble, the available aid is far from satisfactory. Judges and other individuals involved with cases of juvenile delinquency are often unprepared to understand the etiologic and psychologic factors. The preparation of judges, probationary officers, and correction school personnel should contain knowledge and experience with children and their problems as well as study of those conditions in the family, the community, and society which contribute to juvenile delinquency. Law is laudatory, but it is of value only when it helps the citizen.

Children who control anxiety with physical symptoms

Children, in the process of growth and development, are setting up and reenforcing the building blocks of their personalities. In the course of this process, the dynamic ingredients such as security that contribute to the foundation and strength of this structure may be threatened. The consequence is anxiety manifested in behavior symptoms similar to those in adults, as well as in other symptoms peculiar to children. The infant's holding of his breath and the child's temper tantrums and night terrors are evidences of underlying anxiety. Somatic symptoms are also used by children to express anxiety.

A specific event may precipitate an episode of anxiety in a child, but this event is rarely the entire cause of the symptom. Fear of death, anxiety related to a previous illness, or anxiety over a parent's health or welfare may create an underlying anxiety of long duration which can be touched off by a precipitating event. The anxiety attack has many physical components which are frequently evident in cardiac, respiratory, and digestive complaints. Although these attacks are usually temporary, they may return at the occurrence of another precipitating event.

Another manifestation of anxiety is commonly known as hysteria. This condition includes a wide variety of physical symptoms that do not have an organic cause and toward which the individual shows relative emotional indifference. The child's attempt to suppress or repress some painful experience may result in some type of somatic behavior pattern. The range of "hysterical behavior" is wide and difficult to categorize. The symptom may involve the sensory, motor, visceral, and vasomotor functions. Rarely are the somatic manifestations (1) true to the pathologic conditions they resemble, (2) evident when the patient is sleeping, and (3) harmful to the handicapped individual.

The child who develops somatic symptoms, episodic states, or fugues on a hysterical basis is believed to show certain personality characteristics. He often dramatizes his thoughts and feelings. His moods may change rapidly from depression to elation. He is superficial and tends to overimitate and playact. It is not unusual to trace his behavior to a previous experience or the observation of another sick person whose symptoms he has adopted.

Another better organized and more lasting pattern of somatic symptoms may occur in children. The underlying anxiety is usually constant and the cause exists within the environment of the child's everyday life. A child, infected by the parent's control of anxiety by physical symptoms, often adopts this pattern as his. Pleasure and affection gained during illness may make somatic symptoms a blessing in disguise. Unbearable conditions in school or at home may encourage him to seek the solace of illness and invalidism. In other words, the physical symptoms are used by the child to ease the pressures of his anxiety and thus meet needs which are not otherwise satisfied.

Children react in this situation in various ways. Some worry about their symptoms and discuss them constantly. Others delight in it as they give a blow-by-blow account of their aches and pains. Some may not discuss the matter but obviously display the limitations imposed by the symptom. The physical complaints take on a variety of patterns and may simulate to a degree a real physical illness. Headaches, dizziness, weakness, fainting, nausea, indigestion, and constipation are frequent generalized complaints.

The treatment and nursing care of children with this disorder are a very ticklish matter. They are developing patterns of adjustment, and it is important to discourage this behavior. Somatic complaints as patterns of behavior can be fixated or obviated, depending on the wisdom of the treatment plan instituted.

A word on prevention seems apropos. Nurses who care for children in pediatric wards or in other parts of a general hospital should be aware of the dynamics that encourage the development of this pattern of adjustment. Treatment of the whole child rather than of his appendectomy or his tonsillectomy is crucial. Time must be spent with the child if the nurse is to know him and if she is to understand how he feels. The way she allays his fears, the way she prepares him for an operation or treatment, and the understanding and warmth she displays will influence the child's reaction to his illness. The parents' role and their part in helping the child at this time are most important. The nurse is in a position to help the parents by talking with them, by referring them to the physician, and by alerting the physician to the parents' needs.

The child who has developed this behavior pattern is greatly helped by psychotherapy. Given the opportunity, the child will discuss his troubles and soon discover the related causes for his basic anxiety. The somatic complaints quickly disappear since he no longer has any need for them. The part that parents play in the development of this pattern must also receive attention from the therapist.

If the child is hospitalized for his somatic complaints, the nurse should minimize attention to the symptoms, be guided by the psychiatrist's advice, and plan for activities appropriate for the child's age. Reassurance often encourages the child to take a step forward, but the nurse should be alert as to whether she has achieved this encouragement. Sometimes a child cannot accept reassurance any more than can an adult. When the child shows signs of fear or anxiety, the nurse needs to be understanding and provide an adequate explanation to alleviate the fear. Socialization and activities with other youngsters should be very much a part of the planned care. A matter-of-fact attitude toward the physical symptoms is probably better than to ignore them.

Children who control anxiety through ritualistic patterns

The psychodynamics of obsessive and compulsive behavior for children are similar to those for adults. These factors were discussed in Chapter XIV.

Ritualistic activities and play are very much a part of the normal behavior of children. Counting white cars, walking on the line of the pavement, and spitting on the bat for luck are common acts of children at play. However, when the pattern is systematized and permeates the child's daily activities, such as eating and dressing, the behavior becomes a disorder. If the obsessive thoughts and compulsive behavior consume most of the child's waking hours, his school work, and his play, his general health may suffer. Whereas an adult can indulge his obsessiveness and compulsiveness alone, a child often requires and involves other persons. Usually it is the mother who is closest to him and on whom he is dependent for assistance in his daily needs. He imposes on her his repetitious thoughts and demands that she participate in his compulsive acts. This is distressing to the mother, who is usually a rigid, perfectionistic person herself. Her criticism and annoyance add to the child's guilt feelings and to his dilemma. The perfectionism and obsessiveness of the mother or of the father could be etiologic factors of the child's behavior.

Psychotherapy has great value for these children. Primary in therapy are the atmosphere and relationship which provide the child the freedom to talk about his thoughts, feelings, and acts without judgment and ridicule. His parents are too involved and critical of his behavior to provide this need. Understanding and acceptance, regardless of his behavior, are the basis for all relationships with this child. This fact is helpful for the nurse to remember since she, like the mother, may be drawn into the child's pattern of behavior. Patience with respect to the time needed and the peculiar compulsive activity is essential. A plan of daily living, as pleasant and close to normal as possible, should be followed in order to avoid any secondary gains from reenforcement of the ritualistic pattern.

Since obsessive and compulsive tendencies are rooted in parental behavior, psychotherapeutic help for the parents is certainly indicated. Being able to help the mother or father understand and overcome these tendencies is sometimes a difficult project; however, it is vastly important if the child is to be freed of the pattern.

Psychotic behavior in children

In recent years, more investigations and studies have been made of children whose symptoms defy understanding and diagnosis. It is extremely difficult to recognize and detect psychotic behavior in very young children; however, some investigators have reported such findings in infants of less than 1 year of age. Since the life activities of infants and children involve interaction with their environment and principally the people in the environment, it is in this area that signs occur.

Kanner reported in 1944 on early infantile autism in which withdrawal behavior was observed very early in infancy. In the 150 children studied, some common characteristics were detected. The children tended to be self-sufficient, content to be left alone, and ignored the presence of individuals around them. Mothers reported their disappointment when a child did not respond to being picked up. Speech was learned by rote; the child recited poems and words with unusual accuracy, but he lacked the ability to use words to convey appropriate meaning. Autistic children sought to keep things the same and related to objects rather than to people. Their activities were centered around their toys or other objects, and they rarely responded to the persons in the room. Their intelligence appeared to be good, if not superior. And, last, it was recognized that all of the 150 autistic children studied had highly intelligent parents who were interested and preoccupied with their professions or with art rather than with people and their families.

Symbiotic infantile psychosis was described by Mahler in 1952. This condition becomes obvious at a later age than autism. The major symptoms revolve around the intense, close relationship of a child to his mother. The child never learns to relate to other people, and his own identity is lost. The child never separates himself from his mother in identity and proximity.

Since there is so little known about psychotic conditions in children, treatment is equally puzzling. However, each day more knowledge is gained from the investigations and experiences of those persons working with children. Drugs and shock therapy have not been effective. Hopefully, the future will shed more light on the dynamics of these disorders and thus point the way for effective treatment and therapy.

References

Engel, George L.: Psychological development in health and disease, Philadelphia, 1963, W. B. Saunders Co., pp. 29-220.

Freud, Anna: Adolescence. In The psychoanalytic study of the child, vol. 13, New York, 1958, International Universities Press, Inc., p. 255.

Harren, Mary C., Deirelein, Margaret, and Southerby, Verna L.: Residential treatment for the emotionally disturbed child, Journal of Psychiatric Nursing 2:112-126, Mar.-Apr. 1964.

Kanner, Leo: Child psychiatry, Springfield, Ill., 1962, Charles C. Thomas, publisher, pp. 33-172.

Lippman, H. S.: Treatment of the child in emotional conflict, ed. 2, New York, 1962, McGraw-Hill Book Co., Inc.

Mahler, M. S.: On child psychosis and schizophrenia: Autistic and symbiotic infantile psychoses. In The psychoanalytical study of the child, vol. 7, New York, 1952, International Universities Press, Inc., pp. 286-305.

Ohman, Edna N., and Walano, Diane: An appoach to the nursing diagnosis of behavior in the pediatric specialty, Nursing Science 2:152-159, Apr. 1964.

O'Neal, P. and Robins, L. N.: The relation of childhood behavior problems to adult psychiatric states, American Journal of Psychiatry 114:961-969, 1958.

Petrie, Asenath, McCulloch, Rook, and Kasdin, Phoebe: The perceptual characteristics of juvenile delinquents, Journal of Psychiatric Nursing 1:142-151, Mar. 1963.

Chapter XXIV

Nursing care of children with
organic behavior disorders

It has been noted that physical illnesses could be the sources for behavior problems in children, particularly if they result from unsatisfactory parent-child relationships. There are other behavioral changes which are primarily due to organic pathology and secondarily influenced by the parent-child relationship. These organic behavior problems require considerable knowledge and skills in both physical and psychiatric nursing care. The causes for these conditions are numerous and sometimes nebulous. They include congenital anomalies, birth injuries, brain tumors, metabolic and endocrine dysfunction, and infections, to name a few. Invariably children with these conditions require medical care, psychiatric and psychologic guidance, and ingenious nursing care.

The infant in the nursery is routinely examined for his "five fingers and five toes." This examination is a critical point and could mean the initial detection of a neurologic abnormality if the nurse knows and assays the infant's various responses. The infant's period in the newborn nursery should be more than just an automatic feeding, cleaning, sleeping routine. The cry of the infant, his sleep pattern, how he takes his feedings and the amount, and his reaction to individuals are manifestations of his early behavior and should be attentively observed rather than taken for granted.

Congenital anomalies

Congenital anomalies become apparent early in the infant's life, and his development is often marred by some physical deformity and intellectual retardation. Blindness, contractures, paralysis, deafness, and ataxia are commonly observed. The life span of this child is conditioned by the area of the brain involved and the nature of the deformity. The causative factors for malformation of the fetus include hereditary influences, intrauterine complications during pregnancy (Rh factors, toxemias, maternal syphilis, and x-ray of pregnant uterus), and premature birth. Recent reports have also indicated that certain drugs, such as the tranquilizer thalidomide, administered to women during pregnancy could cause the deformity or death of an infant.

Malformation of the brain renders the child, if he survives, intellectually deficient, and, to a greater or lesser degree, dependent on others for his physical needs and daily care. Porencephaly is the absence of part of the brain tissue, sometimes forming a cavity. Death occurs early in infancy. Microcephaly indicates an abnormally small brain and head formation. Hydrocephalus is characterized by an unusually large head due to an increased accumulation of cerebrospinal fluid in the ventricles or subarachnoid space. Infants with these conditions are seen and treated in pediatric nurseries. Their nursing care requires diligent attention to physical needs for the maintenance of health and the prevention of infections since their physical stamina is usually decreased. Although these infants may have a distorted appearance, it is important for the nurse to be aware of and respond to their emotional and psychologic needs which are the same as for other infants. Microcephalic and hydrocephalic children who survive infancy are mentally retarded and require continued detailed care at home, or, as more often occurs, in an institution.

Mongolism is another congenital condition, and is more commonly seen since these children live to the ripe old age of 15 or 16. The mongoloid is conspicuous in his physiognomy and his mental deficiency. His characteristic appearance is marked by a small head flattened posteriorly, eyes with oblique palpebral fissures and vertical folds of skin at the inner canthus, and a flat bridge on a short nose. Other body features are also observable: the limbs are short and the hands are fat and stubby with small fingers, the palms show unusual line markings, the toes and thumbs are abducted from the other digits, and the tongue has deep fissures and often protrudes. Other anomalies may also be present. Mental and physical development is often impaired. The behavior of this child presents very few problems since he is usually cheerful, affectionate, and tends to be obedient. When institutionalized, he adjusts readily and seems content in his environment. He is susceptible to numerous infections, particularly upper respiratory. Although death usually occurs in adolescence, improved medical and institutional care have prolonged life. Depending on his intellectual level, the ability to learn is limited. However, he tends to imitate the behavior of others and takes great pleasure in doing this.

Many of these children, because of their affectionate nature, are dearly loved by their parents and siblings. Consequently they are retained in the home. The increased demand for the mother's time and attention may create problems for the other children. The public health nurse can be of great assistance to the mother and family by her assistance and teaching. There may be day schools for the mentally retarded in the community which would be beneficial for the mongoloid child.

Metabolic and endocrine disorders

Some metabolic disorders, brain tumors, toxic infections, and head injuries result in rapid physical and mental degeneration and inevitable death in a relatively short period of time. Tay-Sachs disease is a hereditary degenerative disease which becomes apparent after the sixth month of life. Its onset is rapid, and the changes, physical and mental, are progressively debilitating and death occurs at about the third year. A cherry red spot on the retina is diagnostic. Muscular weakness and atrophy, blindness, and convulsions, and emaciation, if the child has been inadequately fed, require imaginative and intensive nursing care. Phenylketonuria (PKU) is a disturbance in protein metabolism which is not as devastating as Tay-Sachs and now can be detected and prevented in early infancy. Blood tests for large amounts of phenylalanine and a simple urine test with ferric chloride for urinary phenylpyruvic acid are tests which could signal early treatment and thus prevent brain damage. A low protein diet has proven most therapeutic by reducing the phenylalanine in the blood. Convulsive occurrences and feeblemindedness are major symptoms as the sick child grows and develops. It is common to find several children in the same family afflicted with this disorder, and it tends to be transmitted from parents to children. Early detection in the nursery and by the public health nurse in the home is of primary importance. When the nurse discovers a child with phenylketonuria, she needs to inquire about many, if not all, of the family relatives in order to help prevent the progressive course of this disorder.

Toxic disorders

Brain abscesses, meningitis, and encephalitis may cause brain damage and mental retardation. The toxic factor invades the brain tissues, often causing edema, and, depending on the site involved, results in physical, mental, and emotional changes. The symptoms vary. Drowsiness and lethargy may be present in some patients, whereas hyperactivity and restlessness may be seen in other patients. Vital signs include changes in respiration and pulse and may be observed early. Projectile vomiting and slow pulse and respirations are diagnostic of intracranial pressure, as seen in brain abscesses. As these conditions progress, delirium, convulsions, and coma are serious symptoms. Hallucinations, when they are present, arouse great fear. Constant supervision of these patients is essential to prevent injury, to keep the patients as comfortable as possible, and to observe any changes in their condition. In patients with encephalitis, ocular changes are common, and postencephalitic symptoms often persist due to the original brain damage. These may include changes in the sleep pattern, speech impairment, palsies, tics, ptosis, and convulsions.

During the acute phase of these conditions, the children are very sick and often unresponsive. Their physical care requires extensive medical and nursing procedures to reduce toxicity and to relieve physical discomfort. Nutrition and fluid intake are of primary importance to maintain the child's physiologic needs. When he is immobile for long periods, change in body position alleviates pressure areas. In overactivity, padding the crib or bed helps to avoid injury.

After the acute stage, the child's behavior changes slowly because of the physical exhaustion caused by the disease. An assessment of the physical and mental residual impairments should be a prerequisite for planning his convalescence and rehabilitation. Physical impairments require medical and specialized therapy. Mental impairment and behavioral changes will require psychologic evaluation and psychiatric follow-up.

Personality changes which may result vary considerably with the severity of the illness and the damage incurred. Children who were once well behaved become restless, unruly, aggressive, and explosive. They are difficult to manage at home and at school. Antisocial acts, such as stealing, lying, destructiveness, profanity, and rages may be seen. Although they say they feel remorseful, they also state that they cannot help themselves. Their moods change rapidly, conveying tenderness at one moment and at the next hostility and destructiveness.

Mental growth and intellectual retardation vary with each patient. Some children may suffer no intellectual loss, whereas others may retain the level of achieved development but the development goes no further. And yet other children may lose a great deal of their previous achievment and regress further with time.

Brain tumors and head injuries

Brain tumors are less frequent in children than adults. Head injuries are found more frequently and are caused by birth injuries, falls, accidents, or intentional abuse from parents or siblings. The symptoms of these conditions include headache, dizziness, nausea, projectile vomiting, slow pulse, stupor, and seizures. Specific symptoms are related to the area involved and the size of the tumor or injury to the tissues. Personality changes as prodromal symptoms may be evident to the alert observer. These may include restlessness, irritability, apathy, depression, or confusion to name a few. However, these signs may escape the mother, who sees and accepts variability in the child's daily behavior. It is only when more pronounced symptoms occur that she becomes alarmed. The nurse who may see the child in the doctor's office or clinic may engage the mother in conversation about the child and by so doing identify the onset of gradual behavioral problems or changes. Mental retardation is relative to the pathologic disorder and the success of therapy.

Behavior disorders with convulsions

Fainting, jerking and twitching movements, and convulsions or seizures are not uncommon in children. They may be associated with a physical illness or they may occur spontaneously and without repetition. However, when convulsions are recurrent in children, parents become greatly distressed. They are sure the child is doomed to insanity, mental retardation, or at least moral depravity. It is difficult to erase these ignorant beliefs handed down from the past.

The cause for the convulsions requires serious and thorough investigation. A diagnosis should be made only after careful tests have been taken.

The electroencephalogram is considered the best current diagnostic tool for epilepsy. Once the certainty of idiopathic epilepsy has been established, medication and treatment can be instituted. Most adults with epilepsy experienced its onset in childhood.

Regardless of the cause for the convulsions, there are two attack phenomena observed in children—grand mal and petit mal. The psychic equivalents are rare. The grand mal attacks manifest themselves to a greater or lesser degree in the following manner. An aura or sign may or may not be felt by the child prior to loss of consciousness. Some children give out a shrill cry. The child falls into a tonic spasm making his body stiff and rigid. In a few seconds, clonic movements consisting of twitching, jerking, and kicking movement over the entire body are seen. Mouth and tongue movements and gasping and gargling sounds are exhibited. Tongue biting may occur. The eyes are rolled back and the pupils change from occlusion to dilation. The corneal reflex is absent and the Babinski sign is positive. Involuntary urination and defecation may result. Increased salivation is apparent and sometimes forms a froth on the lips. This stage is followed by relaxation and deep sleep. When the child awakens he may be confused, weak, and drowsy. The child does not remember the attack, but becomes aware that something has happened to him from the manner and facial expression of his parents and others around him. The pattern and regularity of the attacks are not the same, and all attacks do not follow the typical picture just described. Variations among patients and in each individual patient may be observed. The jacksonian-type has specific, characteristic movements, indicating a focal cortical lesion.

Petit mal is used to describe a brief loss of consciousness without seizures. These episodic staring, vacant spells last only a few seconds, and the child is not aware of them at all. A parent, teacher, or playmate may notice the behavior, particularly if they are conversing with the child at the time.

As soon as diagnosis is established, an anticonvulsant medication is usually prescribed to be given. The type and the dosage are dependent on the individual and the ability to control the convulsions. The child's reaction to the medication should be watched carefully, particularly when the drug or dosage is changed or varied. If the drug is discontinued, it is usually done so over a period of time. Some of the more common drugs used are phenobarbital, Dilantin, Mesantoin, Tridione, Paradione, and Phenurone.

A ketogenic diet, containing a low carbohydrate and high fat composition, is more beneficial for children than for adults with epilepsy. The child may find this diet unpalatable unless some imagination and care is used in its preparation. The mother and the nurse may need the expert assistance of a dietitian. Fluids may need to be restricted since some children have shown a decrease in convulsions when dehydration is present.

The child with epilepsy has problems which grow out of the nature of his illness. Parents, siblings, relatives, playmates, teachers, etc., convey some attitude toward the child, particularly when they witness his seizure.

Fear, pity, and revulsion may be portrayed in their faces as their words attempt to mislead the child. It is not unexpected then that the child reacts and thus manifests behavior which may be problematic. This is often interpreted as the epileptic personality. The parental reaction to the child and his condition is vitally important in his adjustment. It must be remembered that these children have similar needs for love, security, acceptance, and happiness as other children. Emotional disturbances have been known to trigger convulsions in some children. Mental deterioration is not a natural concomitant with epilepsy as was once believed. Mental retardation, when evident, is attributed by Lennox to any of five causes: (1) constitutional makeup of the child, (2) injury to the brain before the onset of epilepsy (3) increased frequency of grand mal seizures, (4) toxicity due to overdosage of bromides or phenobarbital, and (5) psychologic and social mistreatment resulting in self-centeredness and severe discouragement. Dostoyevsky, Flaubert, and other persons are witness to the fact that superior intelligence and epilepsy can be compatible. The legendary epileptic personality is a myth rather than a reality.

Nursing care

The nursing care of children generally is not a simple task. Children and their behavior problems are as varied as the individuals. Physical and mental symptoms add to the needs which must be considered in their nursing care. All children have needs which must be met whether at home or in an institution.

The nurse's attitude and knowledge of children, in illness and in health, should result in acceptance of children as they are and in intelligent, creative nursing care. This can happen only if she likes children and has studied their needs. Management of behavior problems requires special attention to child psychiatry and learning experiences with children manifesting behavior problems. The nurse soon realizes that to help the mentally handicapped child she needs the assistance of many other professional and nonprofessional personnel as much as they need hers. It is important that she care for the child and his total needs; therefore she must work, cooperate, and plan with others who are essential for his complete care. If she does not, the child will suffer.

Physical needs. The dependency of children on adults for their physical needs is, of course, related to their age and their physical and mental capacities. When they are sick their dependency is greater. This is particularly true with organic behavior disorders.

The physiologic and medical needs of the child with organic behavior disorders are dictated by the physician. How these are implemented for each child is dependent on the nurse and the child. It is unfortunate that in some instances the nursing care directed toward meeting physical and medical needs is a brisk routine imposed in exactly the same manner on every young patient. The physical and medical care of children requires time and personal involvement.

Comfort aspects for patients with physical abnormalities and behavior disorders require intelligent, imaginative management. The child with cranial and brain trauma may be completely or partially paralyzed, necessitating constant attention. Oral hygiene, skin care, exercise of muscles, and other body movements periodically during the day and night maintain the child's well-being. Management of a child with an enlarged head (hydrocephalus), a paralyzed limb, or total body paralysis (children with Tay-Sachs disease) should be thought through and planned before action is taken. Injury must be avoided. Nurses should instruct and supervise other personnel who assist in the care of these children.

Nutritional needs entail the composition of the diet, the method of preparation, and the manner of feeding. Special diets, such as the ketogenic diet, must contain the nutrients and must be adequate in amount to provide its therapeutic effect. Special and regular diets must be of the consistency for easy ingestion and must be palatable to the child's taste. Appetite is usually poor with illness; nothing should add to this difficulty. Feeding of the child is the direct responsibility of the nurse. The nurse, like the mother, should find the one particular way suitable for feeding each child. Supporting a wobbly head by holding the child in a special position comes with experimentation. The child's swallowing reflex may be impaired, and very small spoonfuls and an adequate length of time at feedings may be required. Tube feeding, when necessary, should include care of the membranes of the nose and the child's general comfort when the tube is inserted or retained in place. The amount of food taken should satisfy the child's hunger as well as maintain his weight and health. Feeding time could be made into a pleasurable experience for the child.

Protection from injury is necessary at all times. The nurse evaluates the environment to see what may be hazardous before any accident or injury happens. The child with convulsions should be in a low bed with a padded headboard if necessary. The spastic child may need constant assistance when walking.

The nurse's responsibility does not end with the child's discharge; she must instruct the mother and sometimes the entire family in how they can best meet the sick child's needs. Referrals to public health nurses for continued care and supervision of this child in the home can contribute much to his well-being and to parents' reassurance.

Psychotherapeutic needs. The child's mental defect is devastating to most parents. Their feelings may be a mixture of guilt, self-pity, revulsion, rejection, and shame. Dealing with parental feelings and attitudes should be started early in order to facilitate acceptance of the child as he is. Only then can the parents and family make a logical plan for his care, growth, and development. Acceptance and understanding are not always achieved and remain a stumbling block in the child's progress. Overprotective parents can also cause harm by fostering overdependency of a trainable child and perhaps by neglecting the other children.

The psychologic needs of these children, as mentioned previously, are the same as for normal children. The parent-child relationship is equally as important. Several authors have written that behavior problems in children with organic brain disorders are stimulated by emotional conflicts growing out of parent or sibling relationships rather than directly from the pathologic disorder. Acceptance and love can go a long way with these children. For the child who is institutionalized, the nurse often becomes the mother figure. Her feelings, attitudes, and behavior toward the child are equally as important as those of parents. Like other children, they benefit by firm but kindly care with an undergird of love and affection.

Since most behavior problems arise within the social and parental relationships of the child, careful study and analysis can detect the true motive underlying the troublesome behavior. Unfortunately, all too often the surface behavior is considered, and the real cause is not unearthed. In young children psychotherapeutic conversations and play sessions help to reveal the underlying problem rather quickly. In older children, it may require more time, closer observations, psychologic testing, and numerous psychotherapeutic sessions. When child-parent relationships are acutely difficult, the removal of the child from home may be best. Hospitalization should then provide the permissiveness for self-expression and acceptance which were lacking in the home. Older children will test the nurse and therapist time and again for their objectivity and true acceptance. The nurse's knowledge of the child's background could be helpful in avoiding pitfalls.

Mental retardation

Mental retardation denotes an impairment in intelligence which is considered lower than average for the individual's level. Impairment may also be observable in maturation, learning, and social adjustment. Retardation varies in degree and in the capacity for mental performance. Severe retardation could render the child a vegatative existence of complete dependence. Some children are less retarded and in a protected environment of a home can develop some training habits for self-care. Still others may be capable of some elementary schooling and job training. The capabilities of each retarded child should be evaluated as one basis for establishing a plan for his development and social adjustment.

Mental retardation has been with man for a long time; however, recent interest and support has brought the matter to the foreground. Research has been stimulated, and resources and facilities have been developed for the care and training of these children. The late President Kennedy's support has given great impetus to this movement. Public education and parent education has helped to change some negative attitudes and the hopelessness which surrounded the mentally retarded. Many patients of all ages who were forgotten in "back-wards" of psychiatric hospitals have been provided with specific facilities for their care and helped to develop whatever abilities they have. Most of the current efforts have resulted in state institutions set up for the care and training of the mentally retarded. Training and education is directed toward the individual's activities of daily living. Many patients are capable of working in the various departments of these institutions under supervision, with the eventual possibility of employment outside.

Community activities have been promoted by parents and by interested citizens. These schools, clinics, and training centers include many volunteers. Special classes in the public school system may be found in some large communities. Financial support for state and community projects is essential to this cause.

References

Blodgett, Harriett E. and Warfield, Grace J.: Understanding mentally retarded children, New York, 1959, Appleton-Century-Crofts, Inc., p. 152.

Casler, Mary Lou: One nurse's approach to understanding and teaching the mentally retarded, Journal of Psychiatric Nursing 2:142-147, Mar.-Apr. 1964.

Davis, Louise: PKU testing in older children, American Journal of Nursing 63:177-178, Mar. 1963.

Dembicki, Eugene L.: Psychiatric drugs and trends—The anticonvulsant drugs. Part I. Journal of Psychiatric Nursing 2:218-222, Mar.-Apr. 1964.

Dembicki, Eugene: Psychiatric drugs and trends—The anticonvulsant drugs. Part II. Journal of Psychiatric Nursing 2:328-330, May-June 1964.

Dunsdon, Emily: Nursing Service in a large institution, American Journal of Nursing 63:75-79, Sept. 1963.

Hilkemeyer, R., Fleming, Ethel B., and Kincaid, Mildred: Nursing care of patients with brain tumors, American Journal of Nursing 64:81-83, Mar. 1964.

Kanner, Leo: Child psychiatry, Springfield, Ill., 1962, Charles C Thomas, Publisher, pp. 267-457.

Leavens, Milam E.: Brain tumors, American Journal of Nursing 64:78-80, Mar. 1964.

Wright, Margaret M.: Care for the mentally retarded, American Journal of Nursing 63:70-74, Sept. 1963.

Appendix

Condensed classification of mental illnesses with diagnostic criteria*

Disorders caused by or associated with
impairment of brain tissue function

I. Acute brain disorders (Chapters 17 and 18†)

Acute brain disorders are due to temporary, reversible impairment of the brain caused by: toxins associated with infection or poisons, circulatory disturbances, neoplasm, trauma, metabolic disturbance, or convulsive disorders. A disturbance in sensorium is the basic symptom syndrome and may be accompanied by hallucinations, transient delusions, and a wide range of behavior changes.

A. Acute brain syndrome associated with intracranial infection.

B. Acute brain syndrome associated with systemic infection.

C. Acute brain syndrome, drug or poison intoxication.

D. Acute brain syndrome, alcohol intoxication.

E. Acute brain syndrome associated with trauma.

F. Acute brain syndrome associated with circulatory disturbance.

G. Acute brain syndrome associated with convulsive disorder.

H. Acute brain syndrome associated with metabolic disturbance.

I. Acute brain syndrome associated with intracranial neoplasm.

J. Acute brain syndrome with disease of unknown or uncertain cause.

K. Acute brain syndrome of unknown cause.

II. Chronic brain disorders (Chapters 17 and 19,)

Chronic brain disorders are due to relatively permanent impairment of the brain. Disturbances of memory, judgment, orientation, comprehension, and affect occur in varying degrees of severity.

A. Chronic brain syndrome associated with congenital cranial anomaly, congenital spastic paraplegia, Mongolism, prenatal maternal infectious disease, and birth trauma.

A secondary mental deficiency superimposed on a chronic brain syndrome.

B. Chronic brain syndrome associated with central nervous system syphilis (meningoencephalitic).

In addition to the symptoms of chronic brain syndrome, will show physical

---

*Summarized from Diagnostic and statistical manual: Mental disorders, published by the American Psychiatric Association Mental Hospital Service, 1785 Massachusetts Avenue, N.W., Washington 6, D. C., 1952.

†Related chapter in text.

signs and symptoms of syphilis, including paretic gold curve. Basic personality orientation (that is, withdrawn, aggressive, etc.) usually exaggerated. Formerly called general paresis.

C. Chronic brain syndrome associated with central nervous system syphilis (meningovascular).
    Mental symptoms usually indistinguishable from the preceding. Suggestive of these categories are early onset after infection, sudden mental changes, focal signs, apoplectiform seizures, very high spinal fluid count, positive blood and spinal fluid serology, and prompt response to systematic antisyphilitic therapy.

D. Chronic brain syndrome associated with other central nervous system syphilis.

E. Chronic brain syndrome associated with intracranial infection other than syphilis.
    May be due to permanent damage resulting from acute brain syndrome.

F. Chronic brain syndrome associated with intoxication.
    Includes incidence of chronic brain damage resulting from lead, arsenic, mercury, carbon monoxide, illuminating gas, drugs, and alcohol. The alcohol group may range from mild to severe, including the chronic delirium classified previously as Korsakoff's syndrome and characterized by polyneuritis.

G. Chronic brain syndrome associated with trauma.

H. Chronic brain syndrome associated with cerebral arteriosclerosis.

I. Chronic brain syndrome associated with circulatory disturbances other than cerebral arteriosclerosis.
    Includes chronic brain damage resulting from cerebral embolism, cerebral hemorrhage, arterial hypertension, and other chronic cardiovascular disease.

J. Chronic brain syndrome associated with convulsive disorder.
    Includes those who show the symptoms of chronic brain damage in association with idiopathic or essential epilepsy.

K. Chronic brain syndrome associated with senile brain disease.
    Includes those senile brain changes ranging from the mild, with self-centeredness, difficulty in assimilating new experience, and labile emotionally, up to the severe, including the state of vegetable existence.

L. Chronic brain syndrome associated with other disturbance of metabolism, growth, or nutrition.
    This group includes Alzheimer's disease (presenile), endocrine disorders, pellagra, disorders associated with avitaminosis.

M. Chronic brain syndrome associated with intracranial neoplasm.

N. Chronic brain syndrome associated with disease of unknown or uncertain cause.
    This group includes familial or hereditary problems such as Huntington's chorea. Others are Pick's disease and multiple sclerosis.

O. Chronic brain syndrome of unknown cause.

III. Mental deficiency
    This category includes primarily those with defects in intelligence existing since birth and without demonstrated organic brain disease or known prenatal cause.

A. Mild: vocational or functional impairment, IQ's approximating 70 to 85.

B. Moderate: require special training and guidance, IQ's approximating 50 to 70.

C. Severe: require custodial or complete protective care, IQ's below 50.

Disorders of psychogenic origin or without clearly defined physical cause or structural change in the brain

Psychotic disorders: characterized by personality disintegration, inability to use reality testing in situations, and inability to relate effectively to other people and to handle own work.

I. Involutional psychotic reaction (Chapter 11.)

Depressions occurring in the involutional period, usually in persons who are compulsive. Typical symptoms are worry, intractable insomnia, guilt, anxiety, agitation, delusional ideas, somatic preoccupation that may become delusional. Depression or paranoid ideas may dominate the reaction pattern.

II. Affective reactions (Chapter 11.)

A severe mood disturbance is primary, with thought and behavior being affected by the mood disturbance.

A. Manic depressive reactions.

Characterized by mood swings, with a tendency to remission and recurrence and may be accompanied by secondary symptoms of illusions, delusions, and hallucinations.

1. Manic depressive reaction, manic type.

Characterized by elation or irritability, circumstantiality, flight of ideas, overactivity. Momentary or transient depression may occur.

2. Manic depressive reaction, depressed type.

Characterized by mood depression, mental and motor retardation, uneasiness and apprehension. Perplexity, stupor, or agitation may occur.

3. Manic depressive reaction, other.

Reactions showing mixture of two preceding, or continuous alteration of the two. Other variants, such as manic stupor or unproductive mania, are included.

B. Psychotic depressive reaction.

A severe depression which includes misinterpretation of reality, differentiated from the manic depressive reaction by the absence of history of previous depressions or mood swings and by the presence of environmental precipitating factors.

III. Schizophrenic reactions (dementia praecox) (Chapters 10 and 12.)

Reactions characterized by disturbances in: reality relationships, concept formations, affective responses, intellectual function, and behavior patterns. Frequent occurrences are strong tendency to retreat from reality, emotional disharmony, stream of thought disturbances, regressive behavior, and, sometimes, deterioration.

A. Schizophrenic reaction, simple type.

Characterized by reduction in external attachments and by impoverishment of human relationships. Apathy and indifference occur. Severity of symptoms increase over a long period of time with mental deterioration. Hallucinations and delusions are infrequent.

B. Schizophrenic reaction, hebephrenic type.

Typical symptoms are inappropriate and shallow affect, silly behavior and mannerisms, giggling, delusions, hallucinations, and regressive behavior.

C. Schizophrenic reaction, catatonic type.

Motor behavior is significant in this group. Generalized inhibition is shown in stupor, mutism, negativism, and waxy flexibility. Excessive motor activity and excitement also occur.

D. Schizophrenic reaction, paranoid type.

The paranoid schizophrenic reaction is characterized by autisic, unrealistic thinking, delusions of persecution and/or delusions of grandeur, ideas of reference, and hallucinations. Behavior is unpredictable, but an underlying hostility and aggression are often constant.

E. Schizophrenic reaction, acute undifferentiated type.

An acute episode that tends to clear, including a wide variety of schizophrenic symptoms. These include confused thinking, emotional upheaval, perplexity, ideas of reference, fear and dream states, and dissociative phenomena.

F. Schizophrenic reaction, chronic undifferentiated type.

Characterized by chronicity and mixed symptomatology of the schizophrenic variety.

G. Schizophrenic reaction, schizo-affective type.
This category includes those who show significant admixtures of schizophrenic and affective reactions.
H. Schizophrenic reaction, childhood type.
Reactions occurring before puberty.
I. Schizophrenic reaction, residual type.
This category includes those who, after a definite psychotic episode, recover sufficiently to get along in the community, but retain evidences of disturbance in thinking, affect, and/or behavior.

IV Paranoid reactions (Chapter 12.)
Characterized by persistent delusions, usually persecutory or grandoise; emotional response consistent with ideas held, and by good intellectual preservation.
A. Paranoia.
A rare disorder characterized by a complex and slowly developed paranoid system usually elaborated logically from a misinterpretation of a real incident. The paranoid system tends to stay isolated and the remainder of the personality is well preserved.
B. Paranoid state.
Characterized by paranoid delusions that lack the logical systematization seen in paranoia. More likely to be of short duration than paranoia.

V. Psychotic reaction without clearly defined structural change, other than above.

Psychophysiologic autonomic and visceral disorders

This group of reactions includes those which represent the visceral expression of affect where the visceral symptoms serve the purpose of keeping the affect from being conscious. This includes what are often called the psychosomatic disorders. There exists a chronic, exaggerated state of normal physiological expression of emotion, with the feeling, or subjective part, repressed. The disorders are characterized by involvement of organs and viscera innervated by the autonomic nervous system and not under voluntary control, failure to alleviate anxiety, physiological rather than symbolic symptoms, and production of structural changes which may be severe enough to threaten life.
A. Psychophysiologic skin reaction.
Neurodermatoses, pruritus, hyperhydrosis, etc., in which emotional factors are important precipitating influences.
B. Psychophysiologic muculoskeletal reaction.
Includes "psychogenic rheumatism," muscle aches and cramps, etc., where emotions are precipitating factors.
C. Psychophysiologic respiratory reaction.
Includes hyperventilation syndromes, bronchial asthma, hiccups, etc., where emotions are precipitating factors.
D. Psychophysiologic cardiovascular reaction.
Includes paroxysmal tachycardia, hypertension, migraine, etc., where emotions are important precipitating factors.
E. Psychophysiologic hemic and lymphatic reactions.
F. Psychophysiologic gastrointestinal reaction.
Includes peptic ulcer, ulcerative or mucous colitis, anorexia nervosa, etc., where emotional factors play a causative role.
G. Psychophysiologic genitourinary reaction.
H. Psychophysiologic endocrine reaction.
I. Psychophysiologic nervous system reaction.
J. Psychophysiologic reaction of organs of special sense.

Psychoneurotic disorders (Chapters 13 and 14.)

These disorders are characterized by anxiety that may be directly felt and expressed or that may be controlled by defense mechanisms such as repression or conversion. Gross distortion of reality does not occur, nor is there gross disorganization of the personality.

A. Anxiety reaction.

Characterized by anxiety that is diffuse and not controlled by defense mechanisms.

B. Dissociative reaction.

A repressed impulse that gives rise to anxiety, with the anxiety controlled by symptomatic expressions, including depersonalization, dissociated personality, stupor, fugue, amnesia, etc.

C. Conversion reaction.

The repressed impulse causing anxiety is converted into functional symptoms, including anesthesia, paralysis, etc. The organs involved are usually under voluntary control.

D. Phobic reaction.

Anxiety is displaced from its original source to some symbolic idea or situation in the form of a neurotic fear. Fear of syphilis, dirt, high places, closed places, and animals are examples.

E. Obsessive compulsive reaction.

Anxiety is associated with the persistence of unwanted ideas or the uncontrollable impulse to commit certain acts. Rituals are carried out despite their unreasonableness to the patient.

F. Depressive reaction.

Anxiety is controlled by depression and self-depreciation.

G. Psychoneurotic reaction, other.

H. All others.

Personality disorders

This category includes disorders that are manifested by a lifelong pattern of behavior rather than by specific mental or emotional symptoms. They include developmental defects or personality trends and are not usually accompanied by marked anxiety or personal sense of distress.

A. Personality pattern disturbance.

Personality types which are almost impossible to alter.

1. Inadequate personality.

Inadequate response evidenced in lack of adaptability, ineptness, poor judgment, lack of physical and emotional stamina, and social incompatibility.

2. Schizoid personality.

Characterized by coldness, aloofness, emotional detachment, fearfulness, daydreaming, quietness, seclusiveness, unsociability, and often eccentricity.

3. Cyclothymic personality.

Characterized by extroversion, personal warmth, friendliness, superficial generosity, alternating moods.

4. Paranoid personality.

Characterized by many traits of the schizoid, along with extreme sensitivity in personal relationships, use of projection, suspiciousness, envy, jealousy, and stubbornness.

B. Personality trait disturbance.

This category includes those with developmental defects that cause them to lose emotional equilibrium under minor or major stress.

1. Emotionally unstable personality.

Excitable and ineffective under stress.

2. Passive-aggressive personality.

Characterized by helplessness, indecisiveness, and dependent relationships, by pouting, stubbornness, procrastination, and passive obstructionism, or by irritability, temper tantrums, and destructiveness.

3. Compulsive personality.
   Characterized by obsessive concern with standards of conscience or conformity, strong inhibitions, inordinate capacity for work, rigidity, and inability to relax.
4. Personality trait disturbance, other.

C. Sociopathic personality disturbance.
   This category includes those whose symptoms are in the area of nonconformity with the cultural standards rather than in the area of personal discomfort and relationships with others.

1. Antisocial reaction. (Chapter 15.)
   Characterized by inability to profit from experience, constant conflict with society, callousness, lack of judgment, emotional immaturity, lack of sense of responsibility, and unusual powers of rationalization. No loyalties.
2. Dissocial reaction.
   Disregard for social codes and conflict with them as the result of an abnormal moral environment. May show strong loyalties.
3. Sexual deviation.
   Includes homosexuality, transvestism, pedophilia, fetishism, and sexual sadism.
4. Addiction. (Chapter 21.)
   Addiction to alcoholism without recognizable underlying disorder; drug addiction.

Transient situational personality disorders

Reactions, transient in character, which appear to a response to situational stress without underlying personality disturbance.

A. Transient situational disturbance.
   For those who cannot be classified otherwise.
B. Gross Stress reaction.
   Ineffective response to overwhelming stress such as fire, earthquake, explosion, etc. The stress may be combat or civilian catastrophe.
C. Adult situational reaction.
   Superficial maladjustment to difficult situation or newly experienced environmental factors.
D. Adjustment reaction of infancy.
   Unusual apathy, excitability, feeding and sleeping problems on a transient basis in infants as a response to interaction with significant persons.
E. Adjustment reaction of childhood.
   1. Habit disturbance: transient habit developed in response to stress, such as thumb sucking, nail biting, etc.
   2. Conduct disturbance: stealing, destructiveness, truancy, etc.
   3. Neurotic traits: reaction manifested primarily as physical and emotional symptoms, such as tics, stammering, phobias, etc.
F. Adjustment reaction of adolescence.
   Transient expression of struggle for independence and vacilliations in regard to impulses and emotional tendencies.
G. Adjustment reaction of late life.
   Transient change in behavior due to physiological, situational, and environmental readjustment.

Glossary

aberration a deviation from what is natural or normal.

acculturation the process by which an individual adapts himself to the culture in which he is reared or adapts himself to another culture.

acute hallucinosis a mental illness associated with the use of alcohol and characterized by auditory hallucinatory experiences predominantly fearful and accompanied by a clear sensorium.

addiction the psychologic and physical dependence upon a drug.

affect A generalized feeling tone distinguished from emotion in being more persistent and pervasive.

aggression a feeling or action that is hostile or self-assertive.

altruism behavior motivated predominantly by an interest in others.

Alzhiemer's disease a condition with marked brain atrophy of a senile type which occurs at an early age period and is characterized by a high degree of dementia.

ambivalence opposing emotions, desires, or attitudes existing at the same time toward an object or person.

amnesia a loss of memory which may vary in length of time or degree of loss.

anxiety a state of apprehensive tension due to real or imagined danger.

apathy a state of indifference in a situation that would ordinarily arouse some response.

attitude a predisposition to react in a manner conditioned by personal endowment and past experience.

autism an introspective absorption in phantasy with a complete exclusion of reality.

behavior deviation behavior which is interpreted as falling outside the accepted limits of the culture.

blocking a sudden stoppage in the stream of thought.

blunting a dullness of emotional response.

childhood a collective term denoting the growth period from infancy to the end of puberty.

compulsion an uncontrollable urge to think or act against one's better judgement.

confabulation the filling in of memory gaps with made-up episodes.

conflict a painful state resulting from the existence of opposing desires, emotions, or goals.

confusion a state of perplexity characterized by lack of clear thinking; in organic states this may include a clouded sensorium.

congruence consistency in thinking, feeling, and actions.

conversion the process by which an emotional conflict is expressed as a physical symptom.

culture the social organization characteristic of a particular group of people.

delirium a state of mental disturbance characterized by confusion, disordered speech, and often hallucination.

delirium tremens delirium induced by prolonged and excessive use of alcohol.

delusion a fixed false belief which cannot be corrected by reason or evidence.

dementia a deterioration of intellectual capacities.

dementia praecox (schizophrenia) a diagnostic term becoming obsolete and being replaced by the term schizophrenia (*see* definition of schizophrenia).

depression a feeling of sadness or dejection.

deterioration an impairment in quality or character.

displacement a mechanism whereby the emotions associated with one idea or object are unconsciously attached to another.

dissociation the detachment of certain aspects or activities of the personality from the control of the individual.

dynamic forceful, active, or in progress.

dynamics of behavior that which impels the patient to behave as he does, the significance and meaning of his behavior, and the purpose of his behavior.

ego the conscious self; that part of the mind which develops to deal with reality.

egocentric self-centered.

electroencephalogram a record or tracing measured by a specific instrument which indicates the rate of electrical discharges in the brain.

electroshock a form of treatment in which a convulsion is produced through the application of electric current to the temporal region of the head.

elopement in psychiatric experience, an escape from the hospital.

emotion a distinctive feeling tone, such as love, hate, fear, etc.

empathy the capacity of feeling in communion with others.

epilepsy a disturbance in consciousness which may be accompanied by convulsive phenomena.

euphoria an exaggerated sense of well-being.

extroversion the direction of interest and emotions toward the environment.

flight of ideas a rapid succession of ideas in which the goal idea is not reached.

functional mental illness a mental illness in which organic change cannot be demonstrated as a consistent accompaniment or cause.

furor a fury or frenzy.

general paresis a syphilitic infection involving predominantly the cerebral cortex.

grand mal a specific convulsive manifestation in which loss of consciousness, tonic spasm, series of jerky movements, and stuporousness follow each other in sequence.

grandiose that which is characterized by affectation, eminence, magnificence, or splendor.

hallucination an imaginary sense perception.

heterosexual sexual attraction for or toward persons of the opposite sex.

homosexual sexual attraction for or toward persons of the same sex.

hydrocephalus a birth defect characterized by an abnormally large head due to an increased accumulation of cerebrospinal fluid in the ventricles or subarachnoid space.

hypochondriasis a morbid preoccupation with the state of health.

hysteria a form of psychoneurosis which includes a wide variety of physical symptoms without organic pathologic changes and toward which the patient shows relative emotional indifference.

id a psychoanalytical term used to denote the unconscious part of the personality which contains primitive urges and desires and is ruled by the pleasure principle.

identification a mechanism by which one feels or thinks as another person.

illusion a misinterpreted sensory perception.

insight a reasonably accurate self-judgment including the emotional acceptance of one's self.

insulin shock a form of treatment in which coma is produced by the injection of sufficient amounts of insulin.

introjection the incorporation and acceptance as one's own of behavior patterns, attitudes, and ideals of others.

introversion the direction of interests and emotions toward one's self.

juvenile delinquency a legal classification of children whose actions and behavior violate the law.

Korsakoff's psychosis a chronic mental illness usually associated with the use of alcohol, characterized by polyneuritis, reduced intellectual capacities, and the marked use of confabulation to compensate for memory loss.

libido a psychoanalytic term meaning the vital force or psychic energy that motivates living.

malinger a deliberate pretense of an illness which does not exist.

manic depressive psychosis a class of mental disorders in which the most dramatic symptoms occur in mood disturbances.

mental mechanism characteristic ways of thinking which serve to meet the needs of the personality.

mental retardation an impairment in intelligence which is considered lower than average for the individual's development.

microcephaly a birth defect involving the formation of an abnormally small head and brain.

motivation that within the individual which prompts him to action.

mutism the inability to speak.

narcissism a phychoanalytic term which denotes self-love.

negativism a generalized resistance to any suggestion from outside the self.

neologism literally, new words.

neurasthenia psychoneurosis in which the predominant pattern is motor and mental fatigability.

neurosis used interchangeably with psychoneurosis; a functional disorder without organic pathology in which the patient's behavior does not seem bizarrely different from the accepted cultural patterns.

obsession the uncontrollable urge to think some thought against one's will.

organic mental illness a mental illness which is accompanied by or caused by organic change.

paranoia a rather rare mental illness characterized by logical and well-systematized delusions of persecution; the personality well preserved.

paranoid same as paranoia; the delusions of persecution less systematized or logical.

perversion a maladjustment in which the sexual object or method of satisfaction deviates from the accepted social patterns.

personality the organization of the sum total of the behavior patterns of the individual.

petit mal a momentary loss of consciousness occurring in epilepsy; muscular twitchings may or may not be present.

phantasy indulgence in daydreaming or fancy usually used in the sense of contrast with reality.

phobia a compulsive fear, or a morbid fear, of an object, situation, or act.

pica the habitual ingestion of substances which have no nutritional value, such as worms, soil, paper, and paint.

pleasure principle the regulation of activity with the purpose of avoiding pain or procuring pleasure.

porencephaly the absence of part of the brain tissue, sometimes forming a cavity.

projection a mental mechanism in which perceptions, motivations, desires, thoughts, and activities, stemming from within the self, are attributed to the external environment.

psychasthenia a form of psychoneurosis in which compulsive patterns of behavior predominate.

psychiatry the branch of medicine which deals with disorders of behavior and personality.

psychoanalysis (1) system of psychology elaborated by Freud which attributes abnormal behavior to repressions in the unconscious; (2) method of treatment designed to investigate the unconscious mental processes.

psychosis mental illness in which the behavior deviations are bizarrely different from the socially accepted standards.

psychotherapy the planned measures undertaken to restore a patient to mental health.

rationalization a mental mechanism whereby the patient substitutes a plausible reason for the real one motivating his behavior.

reaction formation a mental mechanism whereby a character trait is developed to an extreme degree to conceal the presence of its opposite.

reality principle the regulation of activity in accordance with the demands of reality.

regression a mental mechanism whereby an individual reverts to patterns of behavior characteristic of an earlier phase of development.

rejection the act or state of refusing to accept.

repression a mental mechanism which operates unconsciously to keep from awareness unpleasant experiences, emotions, and ideas.

retrospective falsification the distortion of remote memory to fit personality needs.

schizoid resembling or like schizophrenia. This term is usually applied to personalities that are predominantly introverted.

schizophrenia a class of functional mental illnesses characterized by lack of correlation between thinking and feeling and lack of correlation between the patient's experience and reality and with a rich variety of symptoms in thinking, feeling, and motor activities.

> *catatonic type* outstanding peculiarities of conduct with phases of stupor or excitement; latter characterized by compulsive or stereotyped pattern of behavior.
>
> *hebephrenic type* silliness, inappropriateness, bizarre delusions, and hallucinations, appearing early and deteriorating comparatively early.
>
> *paranoid type* form dominated by delusions, especially of persecution and grandeur.
>
> *simple type* apathy, lack of interest, and blunting of emotion with childlike behavior.

self-system the organization of the self with its interrelationships of the organic, the emotional, and the social components; the balance of these interrelationships form the personality orientation which will function to select the elements of experience to which the individual will react.

senile psychoses a group of mental illnesses associated with changes in the nervous system which occur in old age.

sociopathic personality a conduct disorder in which the integration of experience is apparently absent, inhibitory control is reduced, but the intellect remains intact.

stereotypy the use of monotonous repetition of verbal, intellectual, emotional, or motor activities.

stuttering the involuntary hesitation, the repetition of words, or prolongation of sounds in speech.

subconscious that part of the mind which is not immediately focused in awareness but which may be brought to awareness when desired.

sublimation a mental mechanism whereby the energy associated with primitives drives is successfully utilized in constructive social activities.

superego psychoanalytic term used to describe the critical aspect of the personality which is usually equated with the popular term conscience.

suppression a mental mechanism whereby unpleasant feelings and experiences are deliberately kept from awareness.

symbolization the investment of one idea, object, or experience in another.

tic an uncontrollable repetitious gesture or muscular movement.

transference the unconscious identification of another person in a role with which an individual has had past experience.

unconscious that part of mental activity which is not accessible to conscious awareness.

ventilation free verbal expression of feelings, worries, tensions, and problems.

waxy flexibility (cerea flexibilitas) a condition found in catatonic schizophrenia in which the extremities have a waxlike rigidity and will remain for long periods in any placed position no matter how uncomfortable.

Index